NAVIGATING APHASIA

Navigating Aphasia provides the reader with a starting point for working with people with aphasia; presenting key, practical points to consider in the clinical management of this client group.

With a focus on both the language impairment and the consequences of aphasia, this book is packed with easily accessible, applied advice about assessment and therapy from an experienced aphasia clinician. Key sections include:

- Understanding aphasia
- Clinical management
- Assessment
- Approaches to therapy
- Language and cognition
- Living with aphasia.

Concluding with an appendix featuring useful books, websites and professional organisations, this is an essential, practical and comprehensive guide for newly qualified and student speech and language therapists, as well as those new to the world of aphasia.

Tessa Ackerman is a speech and language therapist with over 30 years clinical experience working with adults with aphasia and other acquired disorders of communication. She studied at the University of Leeds, Leeds Polytechnic and the University of York, including postgraduate research on perseveration in aphasia. She has taught undergraduate and postgraduate speech and language therapy students in hospitals, clinics and at universities in the UK. She worked for the NHS for 21 years, including leading a rehabilitation team. For the past 14 years she has worked as an independent speech and language therapist and director of ACT for Yorkshire Ltd. and continues to work with people with aphasia.

NAVIGATING SPEECH AND LANGUAGE THERAPY

Navigating the field of speech and language therapy can seem overwhelming to students and newly qualified therapists. This series is designed to provide concise, entry level summaries of key areas in speech and language therapy, providing a basic insight into a specific area of therapy. Comprising practical advice and guidance from an expert in the field, the books cover topics such as assessment, therapy, psychological approaches and onward referral. This is a useful tool for anyone new to speech and language therapy, or building confidence in their field.

Navigating Aphasia
100 Useful Points for Speech and Language Therapists
Tessa Ackerman

Navigating Speech Sound Disorders in Children
50 Essential Strategies and Resources
Kathryn Murrell

Navigating Trans Voicing
50 Tips, Techniques and Fundamentals for Speech and Language Therapists
Matthew Mills and Natasha Stavropoulos

Navigating Voice Disorders
Around the Larynx in 50 Tips
Carolyn Andrews

Navigating AAC
50 Essential Strategies and Resources for Using Augmentative and Alternative Communication
Alison Battye

Navigating Telehealth for Speech and Language Therapists
The Remotely Possible in 50 Key Points
Rebekah Davies

NAVIGATING APHASIA
100 USEFUL POINTS FOR SPEECH AND LANGUAGE THERAPISTS

Tessa Ackerman

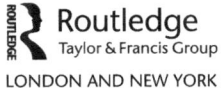

LONDON AND NEW YORK

Cover Image: © Getty Images

First published 2026
by Routledge
4 Park Square, Milton Park, Abingdon, Oxon OX14 4RN

and by Routledge
605 Third Avenue, New York, NY 10158

Routledge is an imprint of the Taylor & Francis Group, an informa business

© 2026 Tessa Ackerman

The right of Tessa Ackerman to be identified as author of this work has been asserted in accordance with sections 77 and 78 of the Copyright, Designs and Patents Act 1988.

All rights reserved. No part of this book may be reprinted or reproduced or utilised in any form or by any electronic, mechanical, or other means, now known or hereafter invented, including photocopying and recording, or in any information storage or retrieval system, without permission in writing from the publishers.

Trademark notice: Product or corporate names may be trademarks or registered trademarks, and are used only for identification and explanation without intent to infringe.

British Library Cataloguing-in-Publication Data
A catalogue record for this book is available from the British Library

Library of Congress Cataloging-in-Publication Data
Names: Ackerman, Tessa author
Title: Navigating aphasia: 100 useful points for speech and language therapists / Tessa Ackerman.
Description: Abingdon, Oxon; New York: Routledge, 2025. |
Series: Navigating speech and language therapy | Includes bibliographical references and index.
Identifiers: LCCN 2024056545 (print) | LCCN 2024056546 (ebook) |
ISBN 9781032199115 hardback | ISBN 9781032199092 paperback |
ISBN 9781003261438 ebook
Subjects: LCSH: Aphasia | Aphasic persons–Rehabilitation | Speech therapy
Classification: LCC RC425 .A25 2025 (print) | LCC RC425 (ebook) |
DDC 616.85/52–dc23/eng/20250524
LC record available at https://lccn.loc.gov/2024056545
LC ebook record available at https://lccn.loc.gov/2024056546

ISBN: 978-1-032-19911-5 (hbk)
ISBN: 978-1-032-19909-2 (pbk)
ISBN: 978-1-003-26143-8 (ebk)

DOI: 10.4324/9781003261438

Typeset in Aldus
by Deanta Global Publishing Services, Chennai, India

To all the people with aphasia I have worked with and their families. Your communication difficulties have taught me about aphasia and the human mind; your courage and fortitude have taught me about the human spirit and how creative and indomitable people can be in their striving to connect. It has been an honour to play a part in your recovery.

"Only connect ... live in fragments no longer."
(E.M. Forster, *Howard's End*)

CONTENTS

Acknowledgements		xii
	INTRODUCTION	**1**

Chapter 1
CAUSES OF APHASIA   4

1	Why is it important to know the causes of aphasia	4
2	Stroke or Cerebral Vascular Accident (CVA)	5
3	ABI (Acquired brain injury)	7
4	Brain tumour	8
5	Dementia	8

Chapter 2
APPROACHES TO UNDERSTANDING APHASIA   11

6	Understanding the brain	11
7	The brain and aphasia	12
8	Neuroimaging and the brain's neural network	13
9	Scans	14
10	Classification of aphasia	15
11	Focus on the language impairment	16
12	Language and cognition	17
13	Language processing models	17
14	Focus on the consequences of aphasia	19
15	A-FROM (living with aphasia: framework for outcome measurement)	20
16	Which approach to use?	21
17	Discussing aphasia with clients	21

Chapter 3
APHASIA MANAGEMENT 25

18	Best practice	25
19	Recovery and prognosis	25
20	Neural plasticity	28
21	Goal setting	29
22	Motivation	32
23	Return to work	33
24	Ending therapy (discharge)	37
25	Measuring outcomes	37
26	Pressures on management	39
27	Brain tumour	39
28	Management at acute stage	40
29	ABI	45
30	Management of chronic aphasia	46
31	Management of progressive aphasia	46
32	Bilingual factors	49

Chapter 4
ASSESSMENT 60

33	Why do we assess?	60
34	Prepare to assess	62
35	Assessment options	63
36	Informal assessment	63
37	Observation	64
38	Semi-structured, interactive interview	65
39	Conversation	66
40	Formal or standardised assessment	71
41	Assessment of language impairment	71
42	Assessment of functional communication	73
43	Assessment as part of therapy	74
44	Impact of assessment	76
45	Some common issues around assessment	77
46	After the assessment	81

Chapter 5
APHASIA AND COGNITIVE IMPAIRMENTS 86

47	Language and cognition	86
48	Executive functions	87
49	Attention	87
50	Memory	88
51	Speed of processing	88
52	Assessment	88
53	Treatments	91
54	Cognitive-communication disorders	93
55	Covid-19	93

Chapter 6
CLINICAL DIAGNOSIS: ASSOCIATED COMMUNICATION DISORDERS 99

56	Apraxia of speech (AoS)	99
57	Dysarthria	102
58	Right hemisphere disorders	105

Chapter 7
TREATMENTS 109

59	Brain stimulation	109
60	Medication	110

Chapter 8
THE THERAPIST, THE THERAPEUTIC RELATIONSHIP AND DIFFERENT ROLES 111

61	What do you need to be?	111
62	The therapeutic relationship	112
63	A supportive environment	112
64	Interactions	113
65	Make connections	114
66	Bring yourself to the therapy session	114
67	Own your expertise	115
68	Share expertise	116
69	Advocate	117

Chapter 9
THERAPY — 120

70	What is it?	120
71	First key steps	120
72	Does it work?	122
73	How much and for how long?	125
74	Limits on provision	126
75	Which therapy?	127
76	Impairment-based treatment – rebuilding and restoring language skills	128
77	Repetition	128
78	Learning	130
79	Examples of impairment-based therapies	131
80	Words for therapy	137
81	Compensatory therapy	137
82	Total communication	142
83	Conversation and support	144
84	Barriers and ramps	146
85	Delivery options	150
86	Aphasia software, computer therapy programs, apps for therapy	154
87	Telehealth	156
88	Therapy gains: generalisation	158

Chapter 10
LIVING WITH APHASIA — 175

89	Impact of aphasia on the individual	175
90	Impact of aphasia on the family	177
91	Living well with aphasia	178
92	A therapy goal	180
93	Adapting the environment	180
94	Public awareness of aphasia	181
95	The psychological impact of aphasia	183
96	The physiological and psychological factors	183
97	Addressing psychological issues	185
98	Assessment of well-being	189

99	Psychological treatments, support and developing strategies	191
100	Looking after yourself: support and development	193

Appendix 1: Framework for outcome measurement (a-from) diagram	203
Appendix 2: Language-processing model	204
Appendix 3: The top ten: best practice recommendations for aphasia (aphasia united "top 10"): international best practice recommendations for aphasia	205
Appendix 4: Some assessments	210
Appendix 5: Useful resources, links and websites	226
Glossary	236
Index	244

ACKNOWLEDGEMENTS

I want to thank the many people who have made this book possible.

My family, who have supported me so much while I was writing it: with special thanks to my husband, Keith, for everything, especially the meals and encouragement and getting everyone we know to ask me, 'Is the book finished yet?' And with thanks to my children, Naomi and Reuben, for advice on how to write and the useful discussions, and for believing I could do it. Thanks are also due to my parents, from whom I learned my love and fascination for language, and to my sister Clare Shephard for her insights. I am grateful to my friends Barbara Power Peretz and Carey Glass for their wisdom across the miles, and for having confidence in me.

My fellow speech and language therapists and friends, Zoe Coates and Frances Haigh. For many years I was fortunate to work with both these wonderful clinicians, and I am grateful for their wisdom and expertise, which helped me to be a better therapist. My thanks too to my former managers and supervisors, Felicity Hudson, Trudy Stewart and Andrew Ellis, for all that they taught me about aphasia and being an SLT. And, lastly, thank you to my friends Claudine Freeman and Sarah Waldram for their advice, and to Jane Madeley of Routledge for her patience.

INTRODUCTION

When writing this book, I thought about what would have been helpful while I was a student speech and language therapist (SLT), and when I started working in the endlessly fascinating and challenging world of aphasia therapy. I had come to SLT from the world of languages; starting with English, Yiddish, French, Latin, Hebrew, then Italian and Arabic. For me, the different words, structures and alphabets were part of the richness, flow and variety of human creativity and connection. When I first read about communication disorders and realised that this connection could be damaged and disrupted, even lost, I wanted to know more. I wanted to understand why, and how, and what could be done to restore what is so essential to all of us.

Language and communication are complex and become more so when they are disrupted. As aphasia therapists, we work with people doing their best to use disordered language systems and navigate their everyday lives. We focus on understanding and treating the language disorder, on improving communication and enabling people to live better with aphasia. Our work is with language, the brain, people, relationships, loss, change, hope and recovery.

Aphasia therapy aims to improve someone's ability to communicate. I find it helpful to think of aphasia therapy as building connections. Connecting and reconnecting. Rebuilding language functions and restoring neural connections. Using remaining language skills to learn new ways to get a message across. Building connections between people; new ones between you, the client and their family, and helping to renew connections between the client, their family and their world.

DOI: 10.4324/9781003261438-1

This book is intended to be a guide to that therapeutic journey of building connections.

Chapter 1 looks at how aphasia is the result of damage to parts of the brain responsible for language processing, and the causes, such as a stroke or brain tumour. The different approaches to understanding and describing aphasia are in **Chapter 2**, including understanding the brain, focusing on language, cognition and language impairment and on the consequences of aphasia with its impact on everyday life. **Chapter 3** focuses on clinical management of aphasia, including best practice, neural plasticity and prognosis, goal setting, ending therapy and the management of acute, chronic and progressive aphasia.

Chapter 4 looks at assessment; why and how we assess, how assessment can be part of therapy, its impact and some common issues. **Appendix 4** has some assessments for reference. People with aphasia can also have cognitive difficulties, and **Chapter 5** looks at language and cognition, some cognitive impairments, cognitive-communication disorders and the post Covid-19 condition. Aphasia is about language and is distinct from other disorders of speech production, **Chapter 6** looks at the associated speech disorders that you will often need to consider and possibly treat alongside aphasia (apraxia of speech, dysarthria).

Chapter 7 touches on brain stimulation and medication as treatments of aphasia that are developing. **Chapter 8** focuses on you, the therapist. It looks at the therapeutic relationship, the different roles you have and shares insights and suggestions based on decades of clinical experience. **Chapter 9** is about therapy. This chapter looks at what aphasia therapy is, and addresses key questions: which therapy, does it work, how much and for how long? There is a focus on both impairment-based treatments and compensatory therapy, while other areas covered include delivery options, software and telehealth.

Chapter 10 looks at the impact of aphasia on the individual and on the family, on living well with aphasia, and how to adapt the environment. **Chapter 11** focuses on the psychological impact and consequences of aphasia, including your role as therapist in supporting your client, and their family and how to look after yourself.

Each section in this book provides references and suggestions of where to go for more information. There is **Appendix 1** with the A-FROM model (Kagan et al. 2008), **Appendix 2** with a language processing model (Whitworth, Webster and Howard 2014), **Appendix 3** gives Aphasia United's international best practice recommendations for aphasia, **Appendix 4** provides examples of aphasia assessments **Appendix 5** has useful links to websites and aphasia organisations that you may find useful.

Experience, study and reflecting on your work will help you to provide more successful therapy, but there is still much that is unknown about aphasia and about how best to treat it. In my experience, it is important to accept and embrace this. Learn from your clients with aphasia, from their perspectives, insights and goals. Learn from other aphasia therapists, and from research into aphasia therapy. Question and evaluate your therapy – ours is a constant learning journey. Remember that what is needed in aphasia rehabilitation is a series of small, planned, incremental steps that can lead to significant achievements. As George Eliot, the Victorian novelist, wrote: "Great things are not done by impulse, but by a series of small things brought together" (Eliot 1859).

REFERENCES

Eliot, G. (1859) *Adam Bede*, Blackwood & Sons, London.

Kagan, A., Simmons-Mackie, N., Rowland, A., Huijbregts, M., Shumway, E., McEwen, S., Threats, T. & Sharp, S. (2008) Counting what counts: a framework for capturing real-life outcomes of aphasia intervention. *Aphasiology*, 22(3), 258–280. https://doi.org/10.1080/02687030701282595

Whitworth, A., Webster, J., Howard, D. (2014) *A Cognitive Neuropsychological Approach to Assessment and Intervention in Aphasia*. Routledge.

Chapter 1

CAUSES OF APHASIA

Perhaps the earliest record of aphasia is in an Egyptian papyrus from around 1700 BCE (Prins & Bastiaanse 2006) where there is a description of someone who had a head injury and 'speechlessness'. However, at that time, people considered the heart to be responsible for the mind (and body) and did not associate the speech problems with the damage to the brain. It was not until the nineteenth century that it was recognised that acquired speech or language deficits were caused by damage to brain tissue (lesions). The work of the aphasiologists Paul Broca (Broca 1863) and Carl Wernicke (Wernicke 1874) highlighted that aphasia is caused by one or more brain lesions in the language-dominant hemisphere. The damage may be focal (localised in one place in the brain) or diffuse (spread over a wider area). Brain lesions can be caused by a stroke (cerebral vascular accident (CVA)), trauma to the brain (acquired brain injury (ABI)), a brain tumour or a progressive neurological disease, including dementia. Because brain lesions can happen at any age, aphasia can affect children as well as adults (an adult is defined here as someone over the age of 18). It tends to be most common in people over the age of 65 because several causes of aphasia, strokes, brain tumours and progressive neurological conditions, tend to affect older adults. This book is aimed at clinicians working with adults with acquired aphasia.

1 WHY IS IT IMPORTANT TO KNOW THE CAUSES OF APHASIA

Causes affect presentation and prognosis and bring different issues to how the aphasia presents, and what your client is dealing with alongside the aphasia. You should understand these and any medical issues your client is dealing with beyond the communication difficulties as they have implications for your clinical management. As speech and language therapists (SLTs) we focus on the language disability, but we know that there are normally other physical and psychological changes as a result of the brain lesions, with resulting mobility and behavioural difficulties adding to the impact on someone's quality of life or life expectancy (see Chapter 10). You also need to be aware of any cognitive and sensory difficulties someone may have as a result of, e.g. an acquired brain injury, such as attention and memory difficulties.

Knowing about the medical background of your client includes understanding the nature and site of the brain lesions caused by, e.g. the tumour, the physical and cognitive issues they are dealing with, the medical treatments and any side-effects and the prognosis. The damaged areas (lesions) are normally seen on a diagnostic imaging scan, and you should find details in the medical notes. You will need to read the medical notes and scans carefully, ask your colleagues questions if you do not understand the information in the notes or scan, and ask the client and their family what they have been told. Re-read your anatomy textbooks, familiarise yourself with reading scans. An aphasia therapist should make themselves well-informed because part of your therapeutic role is to help your client and their family understand the aphasia better, and you should be familiar enough with the causes of their aphasia to answer their questions or know where to find the answers.

2 STROKE OR CEREBRAL VASCULAR ACCIDENT (CVA)

A stroke or cerebral vascular accident (CVA) occurs when the supply of blood and oxygen to part of the brain is interrupted or reduced, resulting in focal lesions in brain tissue. There are two types of strokes: an ischaemic stroke (also called a cerebral infarct) which occurs when the blood vessels are blocked; and a haemorrhagic stroke, when blood vessels leak. Around 85 per cent of strokes are **ischaemic strokes**. Common causes of a blockage include narrowing of the arteries (atherosclerosis) or a blood clot (embolism) which blocks a blood vessel. The blood supply is reduced and with it the oxygen and nutrients needed to keep brain tissue alive. Our arteries may become narrow with age, or as a result of high blood pressure (hypertension), due to high cholesterol, diabetes, obesity, smoking and high alcohol intake. A family history of stroke is also a risk factor. The other 15 per cent of strokes are **haemorrhagic strokes** involving bleeding into the brain (also called an intracerebral haemorrhage). Bleeding can be caused by the rupture of a blood vessel (after the wall of a blood vessel weakens or thins). Sometimes the weakened wall swells, causing a bulge called a brain or cerebral aneurysm; this can then burst, and blood leaks into the surrounding area of the brain. An abnormal connection between arteries and veins (an arteriovenous malformation) can also rupture. The main cause of haemorrhagic strokes is hypertension (and the risk of this increases with smoking, drinking heavily, being overweight and a lack of exercise). After a stroke, there may be a further, diffuse brain injury due to oedema (swelling), haemorrhage (bleeding), anoxia (loss of oxygen supply) or infection. A **TIA** (**transient ischaemic attack**), sometimes called a 'mini-stroke', involving a temporary period of symptoms similar to a stroke, does not result in brain lesions. It can be a sign that someone may have a stroke; with one in three people who have a TIA going on to have a full stroke.

People with aphasia and their family often ask whether they might have another stroke. This can be the cause of part of the increased anxiety experienced (see Chapter 10, points 95 and 96). You will need to judge how much information to give when they ask, and how to do so. Normalising the question can be helpful; you could begin a conversation with, 'many people who have a stroke are concerned ....' observe their reactions and let that guide you. It is helpful to use written information which covers the warning signs, causes and risk factors for stroke (see Further Reading); have the information visible to everyone, highlight and read aloud key words and use the pictures and diagrams to support the conversation; taking care to answer questions, give clients information to take away with them and refer them to other health care professionals for further advice. Revisit the conversation again, as required; how much information people are able or willing to take in varies from person to person; both someone with aphasia and their family members. Don't assume that once it has been discussed, the job is done.

3 ABI (ACQUIRED BRAIN INJURY)

Acquired brain injury (ABI) may be the result of a trauma (so it is often called a traumatic brain injury (TBI)); following a road traffic accident, a fall (e.g. while playing a sport, or at home); an assault or following surgery to remove a brain tumour. The TBI may be closed (no skull fracture) or open (e.g. bones from the skull fracture penetrate the brain). An ABI can result in both focal and diffuse brain injuries. Focal injuries may involve lacerations, or tears to the brain tissue. These can lead to intracranial haematoma (blood collecting in the skull). The injuries may involve contusions (small haemorrhages) often at the tips (or poles) of the frontal, temporal and occipital lobes. Following a TBI, there may be a further diffuse brain injury due to oedema, haemorrhage, anoxia or infection. **Anoxic brain injury**: the brain is highly sensitive to any reduction in oxygen supply and when there is lack of oxygen neurons begin to die within minutes. Anoxic brain injury can occur following a stroke or TBI. It may also occur following a heart attack, as a result of suffocation (e.g. in a fire), strangulation, near drowning, a respiratory arrest (e.g. following drug overdose). **Other causes of brain injury** may be metabolic/toxic (e.g. renal failure, carbon monoxide poisoning). Some infections can damage the brain (e.g. meningitis) and there are very rare autoimmune causes of brain injury (e.g. autoimmune encephalitis).

4 BRAIN TUMOUR

There are over 100 types of brain tumour, which can start anywhere in the brain or in the spinal cord, causing different symptoms depending on where they are located. Brain tumours can be benign and grow slowly. Meningiomas are the most common type of primary brain tumours, they are usually benign and develop slowly. If cancerous, brain tumours are either primary (begin in the brain) or secondary/ metastatic (the cancer spreads to the brain from other parts of the body). The most common type of cancerous (malignant) brain tumour in adults is a glioblastoma. While not all brain tumours are life-threatening, they can cause problems for normal brain functioning, e.g. by invading and destroying healthy brain tissue, putting pressure on nearby brain tissue or increasing intracranial pressure and causing bleeding in the brain. People can then have symptoms including aphasia and problems with memory, vision, balance or walking. Common treatments for brain tumours include surgery and radiation therapy. The brain surgery to remove a tumour can result in complications including brain lesions around the site of the tumour. Communication impairments can be among the most frequently reported long-term consequences of a brain tumour, both before and after surgery (Milman et al. 2020, Finch & Copland 2014).

5 DEMENTIA

Dementia is a neurodegenerative disease and involves the loss of neurons and atrophy in parts of the brain, leading to a progressive and persistent decline in cognitive functioning, including language and memory. The impairments limit someone's participation in work, activities of daily living (ADL) and ability to communicate. There are different types of dementia. Alzheimer's dementia (AD) with an insidious onset and gradual progression. Vascular dementia (VaD) reflects the vascular events causing it, often with a stepwise deterioration of symptoms. Dementia with Lewy bodies (DLB) and Parkinson's disease (PD) with dementia also involve neurodegenerative disorders. There are 'mixed' dementias with features of AD and VaD or features of AD and DLB. Frontotemporal lobar degeneration (FTD/FTLD) and progressive aphasias involve a progressive loss of language. See Chapter 3 regarding the areas of the brain affected and implications for speech and language deficits. See Chapter 9 for management of primary progressive aphasia (PPA).

REFERENCES

Broca, P. (1863). Localisation des fonctions cérébrales. Siège du langage articulé. *Bulletins de la Société Anthropologique de Paris* (séance du 2 avril), 200–204.

Finch, E., & Copland, D. A. (2014). Language outcomes following neurosurgery for brain tumours: a systematic review. *NeuroRehabilitation*, 34(3): 499–514. https://doi.org/10.3233/NRE-141053

Milman L., Anderson E., Thatcher K., Amundson D., Johnson C., Jones, M., Valles, L., & Willis, D. (2020). Integrated discourse therapy after glioblastoma: a case report of face-to-face and tele-neurorehabilitation treatment delivery. *Frontiers in Neurology*, 11: 583452. doi: 10.3389/fneur.2020.583452. PMID: 33329328; PMCID: PMC7710897.

Parr, S., Pound, C., Byng, S., & Moss, B. (2004). *The Stroke and Aphasia Handbook*. Connect Press.

Prins, R., & Bastiaanse, R. (2006) The early history of aphasiology: from the Egyptian surgeons (c. 1700 BC) to Broca (1861), *Aphasiology*, 20(8): 762–791. doi: 10.1080/02687030500399293

Wernicke, C. (1874). *Der aphasische Symptomencomplex: Eine Psychologische Studie auf Anatomischer Basis*. Cohn & Weigert.

FURTHER READING

Atkinson, M. and McHanwell, S. (2018). *Basic Medical Science for Speech & Language Therapy Students*, 2nd ed. J&R Press Ltd.

Gage, N. M. and Baars, B. J. (2019). *Fundamentals of Cognitive Neuroscience A Beginner's Guide*, 2nd ed. Academic Press.

Papathanasiou, I., Coppens, P. (2022). *Aphasia & Related Neurogenic Communication Disorders*, 3rd ed. Jones & Bartlett Learning.

Parr, S., Pound, C., Byng, S., & Moss, B. (2004). *The Stroke and Aphasia Handbook*. Connect Press.

Seikel, J. A., Drumright, David G., & Hudcock, Daniel J. (2021). *Anatomy & Physiology for Speech, Language, and Hearing*, 6th ed. Plural Publishing.

Chapter 2

APPROACHES TO UNDERSTANDING APHASIA

6 UNDERSTANDING THE BRAIN

Providing information about the nature and impact of the brain lesion can be an important start to someone's aphasia therapy and recovery. While your client knows that something has happened to affect how they communicate, many will have little knowledge of the brain, or even connect the two. It can be helpful, even empowering, for people to understand something about what the brain does and how it works to provide a context for what has happened. Start by checking what they know. Use diagrams, pictures, drawings and key written and spoken words. Simplify the concepts. See Further Reading for suggested books and websites. Depending on the client, you could give them information about:

- The brain and the central nervous system: the cerebrum, the brain stem and the cerebellum, the spinal cord.
- The way the cerebrum divides into two (cerebral) hemispheres and has four parts or lobes: the frontal, temporal, parietal and occipital lobes.
- The cerebral cortex (surface layer of the cerebrum), with billions of tightly packed neurons (nerve cells: the grey matter of the brain, key for processing information. (If relevant to the client, mention the basal ganglia, thalamus and hypothalamus within the cerebrum.) How, in order to increase the surface area of the cerebral cortex, it is packed tightly into folds (gyrus/gyri) and grooves (sulcus/sulci) or

fissures. These make the boundaries between the lobes and hemispheres.
- The vascular system and blood supply of the brain and how the brain needs the oxygen and glucose from the blood to function.

7 THE BRAIN AND APHASIA

Relate your client's brain lesions and experiences to the model of the brain. They may already know something about what has happened and may want you to explain terms or words, e.g. a middle cerebral artery (MCA) stroke. This is likely to be a common question as the MCA is the most common artery involved in acute strokes and supplies areas including the frontal, temporal and parietal lobes. It is helpful to use the generalisation: 'acquired aphasia results from damage to left-hemisphere temporal, frontal, and parietal brain regions that are critical for language' (Kertesz et al. 1979). And to say that when the damage is in these parts of the brain, it is likely that several different language abilities will be affected. Make the link between the brain lesion and the changes in communication.

Many of the people you work with after an **acquired brain injury (ABI)** may present with anoxic brain injury which causes diffuse damage to many areas of the brain, and a range of language and cognitive difficulties (see Chapter 5). They may have injuries to the brainstem leading to difficulties with cognitive skills including memory and language as well as ataxic dysarthria, a motor speech disorder (see Point 57) (Zhang et al. 2023).

Brain tumours cause problems with normal brain functioning by destroying healthy brain tissue, putting pressure on other areas of the brain, increasing intracranial pressure and causing bleeding in the brain. The impact on brain function can lead to physical and cognitive problems, e.g. with balance, walking, memory, vision and aphasia. There is more likely to be aphasia when the tumour is in the left hemisphere of the brain, particularly in the frontal and/or temporal lobes.

Dementia involves a loss of brain tissue function and permanent cognitive impairment. Alzheimer's (AD) involves the temporal, parietal and frontal lobes. Vascular dementia (VaD), or vascular cognitive impairment (VCI), often involves widespread vascular lesions with a progressive decline in cognitive and language functions. Frontotemporal lobar degeneration (FTD/FTLD) involves the frontal and temporal lobes and includes primary progressive aphasia (PPA) where there is a progressive loss of language abilities. PPA is classified into three types: progressive non-fluent aphasia (PNFA); semantic dementia (SD); and logopenic progressive aphasia (LPA). See Chapter 9 for more on PPA.

Most people with aphasia want to tell the story of the stroke or TBI, if they can do so and/or have a clear memory of the event. Some people need or want their family to tell the story for them, beginning with the first signs of the stroke or brain tumour, or how the brain injury occurred. Perhaps they collapsed, had weakness or paralysis in the face, arm or leg; slurred or unintelligible speech and/or difficulty understanding what was said to them; double vision or balance problems. They may be continuing to experience all or some of these difficulties. They may have other issues, such as emotional lability (uncontrolled crying or laughing), fatigue, seizures, incontinence, pain, limb apraxia, depending on where in the brain the lesions occurred. Listen attentively to this account. Not only do you hear important information about the medical history, but you have an example of someone's communication attempts, perhaps some speech, and you start to see the impact of the aphasia; are they frustrated, silent? You may also see how both the person with aphasia and their family are managing the changed communication in conversation.

8 NEUROIMAGING AND THE BRAIN'S NEURAL NETWORK

Beyond the site of lesion(s), neuroimaging has highlighted that language functions use a network that involves the frontal, temporal and parietal regions of both hemispheres of the brain, working together as a whole, with an interactive neural network: 'speech and language processes depend on the integrity of the entire network comprising both cortical structures and their interconnected fibre tracts' (Døli et al. 2021). So, aphasia is caused by damage to individual areas of the brain and to this complex neural network responsible for language processing. Understanding someone's aphasia benefits from knowing which area(s) of the brain have been damaged and what the language profile (level of skills and deficits in speech, writing, reading and understanding) suggests about the damage to the neural network.

9 SCANS

Your client may have various scans and may want to know why they are having them, what they are for and what they involve. You can explain these to clients using pictures and words (see Further Reading).

- CT or CAT scan: (computerised tomography or computerised axial tomogram) uses X-rays to generate two-dimensional images of slices of the brain (or body). It can see whether there has been a cerebral infarction (an area of brain tissue that has been damaged due to a thrombus or embolus obstructing the blood supply), or a haemorrhage (a blood vessel in the brain has leaked into the surrounding tissue).
- MRI (magnetic resonance imaging) makes use of the magnetic properties of organic tissue to generate brain images using magnetic waves. It provides a sharper image of bone and soft tissue, contrasts grey and white matter and is better than a CT at spotting more subtle lesions.
- fMRI (functional magnetic resonance imaging) uses MRI imaging techniques while someone is performing a task to measure levels of neural activity, in this way the scan can identify which regions of the brain are activated when someone is carrying out a cognitive activity.

- PET (positron emission tomography) scans measure physiological function by looking at e.g. blood flow and oxygen consumption in different parts of the brain. An area of tissue damage (from e.g. a brain tumour) would have poor blood flow.

10 CLASSIFICATION OF APHASIA

Your client and their family may have been told that the client has 'Broca's' or 'receptive' or 'expressive' aphasia. These terms come from classification systems (Anderson et al. 1999) including the Boston School which separates aphasia into eight subtypes of aphasia, according to a set of symptoms and lesion sites: 1) Broca's, 2) Transcortical Motor, 3) Global, 4) Mixed Transcortical, 5) Wernicke's, 6) Transcortical Sensory, 7) Conduction and 8) Anomic. It is useful to be aware of the terminology because these terms are used by other health professionals and in aphasia literature, particularly:

- **Broca's aphasia:** Broca called the left posterior inferior frontal gyrus the 'speech centre' and suggested that damage in this area lead to 'non-fluent' or 'expressive' aphasia; with good comprehension, poor spontaneous speech, poor naming and repetition.
- **Wernicke's aphasia:** Wernicke suggested that damage to the left posterior, superior temporal gyrus was responsible for what is referred to as 'fluent' or 'receptive' aphasia, with spontaneous speech that is fluent but lacking in meaningful content, with non-word errors, difficulties with auditory and reading comprehension, poor naming and repetition.
- **Global aphasia:** refers to aphasia that has a significant impact on all aspects of communication, with poor auditory and written comprehension and poor production of spoken/written language, poor spontaneous speech, poor naming and repetition.

The syndromes in classification systems do not correspond to specific brain lesion sites and only 30–40 per cent of people with aphasia fit neatly into the classifications (Selnes 2001). So, a client labelled as having Broca's aphasia may have relatively intact auditory comprehension and limited speech production, but you will find that most people with aphasia do not neatly follow the descriptions of a category and that the label does not help you work out appropriate therapy.

So, with classifications not providing a useful basis for therapy, our diagnosis and treatment of people with aphasia more usefully learns from approaches focusing on language, cognition, communication and the consequences of aphasia.

11 FOCUS ON THE LANGUAGE IMPAIRMENT

It is helpful to start with the World Health Organisation's *International Classification of Functioning, Disability and Health (ICF)*, (WHO, 2001). This highlights how an impairment interacts with the environment to affect functioning in the world. It provides a framework to approach aphasia, including all the key areas: the brain lesions, damage to language processing and cognition, the impact on everyday life and the communication disability it can bring. There are different levels of aphasia:

- Body functions and structures (impairments of the brain and functions of the brain: language and cognition)
- Activity (everyday behaviours and activities that require the use of language to communicate, using four modalities – understanding, speaking, reading and writing)
- Participation (the importance of communication for involvement in everyday life; work, relationships and social life)
- Environment (attitudes of other people to aphasia, barriers to participation in the world).

12 LANGUAGE AND COGNITION

Linguistic concepts and rules help us describe and understand the disordered language of aphasia, and its impact on communication. We can look at which linguistic processes and rules are being used appropriately and which are disordered, e.g. speech production in terms of phonology and phonetics, non-verbal communication such as gesture. Cognitive neuropsychology focuses on how cognitive skills including understanding and producing language are organised in the brain. Aphasia is seen as caused by impairments to parts of the language processing system and to the connections between those parts.

13 LANGUAGE PROCESSING MODELS

Language processing models help to visualise this system, including logogen models. The logogen model commonly used (see Appendix 2) has boxes and arrows: where the boxes represent the different language processes, and arrows represent the connections between the processes. Each component of the model is needed to process a single word. We make certain assumptions about the way the system works. Some of the boxes operate independently (they are modular). Some can be localised to a particular part of the brain, so brain lesions can damage or destroy one or more boxes (processes) and/or the arrows (connections) between them. Everyone presents with the same underlying language processing system that is represented by the logogen model. With aphasia, we are working with a system that has been damaged with one or more language skill(s) impaired or removed. The parts of the system that are unimpaired can be used in a new way, e.g. someone with acquired dyslexia, who can only read a word by spelling it out letter-by-letter, is using their unimpaired ability to recognise a word that is spelled out loud to them to read the word.

This theoretical model (Patterson & Shewell 1987) is useful to clinicians because the language of someone with aphasia may seem chaotic and unfathomable, but there are patterns to the disordered language of aphasia, which follow the underlying structure and rules of the language processing system. It accounts for the dissociations we see (when someone can understand a word that they read, but not understand the same word in spoken form, for example, or the other way around). Assessments that use the logogen model help us build detailed descriptions of someone's language deficits (see Chapter 4) and create individual profiles of where the difficulties are in their language system, which processes and connections have been damaged and account for the specific language difficulties they are experiencing. Which components and their connections are impaired varies from one person with aphasia to another, so no one you treat will have the same presentation. The model does not tell us everything we might want to know about what is going on in the boxes or between them, but it remains a vital part of our clinical approach to aphasia because it helps us identify the nature of the language problems, assess them and design treatments.

There are other models that try to explain the complex language breakdown in aphasia. Neuroimaging suggests that the brain handles information with interactive processing; whereby cognitive processes are carried out by neural networks that are bidirectional (function in two directions). Interactive activation models show this bidirectional interaction between units that encode information such as phonemes, letters or words. The triangle model is a computational model of word processing which suggests three language systems (semantics, phonology and orthography) and three bi-directional pathways to both understand and produce language, so there are no lexicons as in the logogen model (Seidenberg & McClelland 1989). In this model, the semantic, phonological and orthographic information needed to produce or understand a word is processed simultaneously (Madden, Torrence & Kendall 2020). Processing a word involves activation across processing units that connect into complex networks. These models are currently unable to account for the dissociations between language skills which we see in people with aphasia (in the way the logogen model can). They may add to our understanding of aphasia in the future but currently are less helpful to us when trying to understand the underlying language difficulties of the client in front of us.

Of course, no model can explain everything about aphasia. Cognitive neuropsychology builds the models using data from normal language processing and the language of people with aphasia and with ongoing research using this data, revising and improving the theories behind the models. Cognitive neuropsychology's approach to aphasia has been invaluable in helping us to address key issues about the language difficulties of our client with aphasia. It provides assessments that give us a detailed language profile, which in turn points to impairment-based therapy and to measuring outcomes of therapy. In clinic, you can use diagrams of models to explain the rationale for any impairment-based therapy you may suggest. You can find models in some published assessment instructions, e.g. PALPA (Kay, Lesser & Coltheart 1992), and therapy resources. Sharing these can be helpful; a visual representation, where the aphasia is out in the open, down on paper and something understood, put in a context, shared by others and not just an individual's problem. You can draw your own, simplified versions of models, too.

14 FOCUS ON THE CONSEQUENCES OF APHASIA

Aphasia is a language impairment with consequences on someone's ability to participate in activities and the world around them. In this sense, it is a life-changing event (Duchan & Byng 2004) because communication difficulties have a negative impact on so much of someone's life. The focus is not on restoring language function, but on compensating for the aphasia to improve communication, with therapy aiming to reduce the negative consequences of the aphasia.

15 A-FROM (LIVING WITH APHASIA: FRAMEWORK FOR OUTCOME MEASUREMENT)

To understand the consequences that aphasia has on someone's communication, it is useful to use the Living with Aphasia: Framework for Outcome Measurement (A-FROM) (Kagan et al. 2008), see Appendix 1. This is a model that translates the *ICF*(WHO, 2001) into a framework for measuring the impact of aphasia. It focuses on how aphasia affects someone's ability to engage in everyday communication activities and in social interaction. It offers a framework for understanding and treating aphasia and is a helpful model to use with clients when discussing what aphasia is, its impact on everyday life, goals and therapy options. In this social model of aphasia, the focus is on aphasia as a communication disability ('A physical or mental impairment that has a substantial, adverse, and long-term effect on your ability to carry out normal day-to-day activities').[1] This approach highlights that there can be a difference between the impairment someone has and the disability it causes. A lack of speech, due to an impairment of spoken word production, becomes a significant disability for someone with aphasia if they have no other way of getting their message across. If they have access to pen and paper to use writing and drawing and a conversation partner to meet their communication attempts with knowledge of aphasia and of supported conversation, the aphasia is less of a barrier to communicating their thoughts and wishes.

So, people with aphasia are unable to participate in an environment that does not enable access to someone with impaired communication; it is the environment that makes the aphasia more disabling than it needs to be. The focus is then on making the environment aphasia-friendly. Someone's immediate environment might be their family and friends. There is a lack of understanding of aphasia in the wider world, which means that people with aphasia face barriers to participating in work and wider social life because of their communication disability. The Life Participation Approach in Aphasia (LPAA Project

Group 2001) provides a model of how it is possible to educate the community around someone with aphasia, with an emphasis on a shared responsibility for the success of communication (see Chapter 10).

16 WHICH APPROACH TO USE?

As clinicians, we focus on how the different approaches and models can help us to address whatever the client with aphasia brings. We need to be knowledgeable about the different approaches, flexible and eclectic and offer a wide range of therapy options and techniques to work towards our client's goals. Many, if not most, therapy interventions combine different approaches, using the A-FROM and language processing models to offer therapy that addresses the impairment and consequences of aphasia. For example, with a goal of increasing participation in chosen conversations, someone may work on improving the ability to produce a set of spoken words in a specific environment along with strategies to manage any word retrieval difficulties and educate and involve other people around them to provide support (see Mrs. B in Chapter 10).

17 DISCUSSING APHASIA WITH CLIENTS

As well as using diagrams and models, it is helpful to use metaphors, with pictures and spoken and written words to talk about what aphasia involves. For example, explaining word retrieval difficulties, you could use a picture of a library where books have been thrown off the shelves, or a filing cabinet with the papers and files strewn on the floor. The books and files represent words being disorganised, still somewhere but inaccessible or difficult to find. People who begin a sentence and come to an abrupt halt can appreciate the metaphor of a motorway with roadworks and traffic jams. This can be extended to using the idea of coming off the motorway, down slower roads to get to a destination when working on alternative ways of getting a message across, such as circumlocution or combining non-verbal and verbal strategies. When discussing aphasia, include an introduction to rehabilitation. Give some initial information about the nature of recovery and of rehabilitation and therapy (see Chapters 7 and 10) with a view to helping someone appreciate why you encourage regular, repetitive practice of a language skill or why it is helpful for them to look beyond speech to get their message across.

NOTE

1 Definition from the Equality Act, UK 2010.

REFERENCES

Anderson, J. M., Gilmore, R., Roper, S. et al. (1999). Conduction aphasia and the arcuate fasciculus: a re-examination of the Wernicke–Geschwind model. *Brain and Language*, 70(1):1–12. doi: 10.1006/brln.1999.2135.

Døli, H., Helland, W. A., Helland, T., & Specht, K. (2021). Associations between lesion size, lesion location and aphasia in acute stroke. *Aphasiology*, 35(6): 745–763, doi: 10.1080/02687038.2020.1727838

Howe, T. J., Worrall, L. E, & Hickson, L. M. H. (2008). Observing people with aphasia: environmental factors that influence their community participation. *Aphasiology*, 22(6): 618–643. https://doi.org/10.1080/02687030701536024

Kagan, A., Simmons-Mackie, N., Rowland, A., Huijbregts, M., Shumway, E., McEwen, S., Threats, T., & Sharp, S. (2008). Counting what counts: a framework for capturing real-life outcomes of aphasia intervention. *Aphasiology*, 22(3): 258–280. https://doi.org/10.1080/02687030701282595

Kay, J., Lesser, R., & Coltheart, M. (1992) *Psycholinguistic Assessments of Language Processing in Aphasia (PALPA)*. Lawrence Erlbaum Associates.

Kertesz A., Harlock W., & Coates R. (1979). Computer tomographic localization, lesion size, and prognosis in aphasia and nonverbal impairment. *Brain and Language*, 8(1): 34–50. doi: 10.1016/0093-934x(79)90038-5. PMID: 476474

Laine, M., & Martin, N. (2012). Cognitive neuropsychology has been, is, and will be significant to aphasiology. *Aphasiology*, 26(11):1362–1376. https://doi.org/10.1080/02687038.2012.714937

Madden, E. B., Torrence, J., & Kendall, D. L. (2020). Cross-modal generalization of anomia treatment to reading in aphasia.

Aphasiology, 35(7): 875–899. https://doi.org/10.1080/02687038.2020.1734529

Patterson, K., & Shewell, C. (1987). Speak and spell: dissociations and word-class effects. In M. Coltheart, G. Sartori, & R. Job (Eds.), *The Cognitive Neuropsychology of Language* (pp. 273–294). Lawrence Erlbaum.

Plaut, D. C., McClelland, J. L., Seidenberg, M. S., & Patterson, K. (1996). Understanding normal and impaired word reading: computational principles in quasi-regular domains. *Psychological Review,* 103(1): 56–115. doi:10.1037/0033-295X.103.1.56

Sarno, M. T. (1997). Quality of life in aphasia in the first poststroke year. *Aphasiology,* 11(7): 665–679. https://doi.org/10.1080/02687039708249414

Seidenberg, M. S., & McClelland, J. L. (1989) A distributed, developmental model of word recognition and naming. *Psychological Review,* 96(4): 523–568. doi: 10.1037/0033-295x.96.4.523.

Selnes, O. (2001). A historical overview of contributions from the study of deficits. In B. Rapp (Ed.), *The Handbook of Cognitive Neuropsychology: What Deficits Reveal about the Mind* (pp. 23–41). Taylor & Francis.

Wernicke, C. (1969). The symptom complex of aphasia. In R. S. Cohen & M. W. Wartofsky (Eds.), *Proceedings of the Boston Colloquium for the Philosophy of Science 1966/1968. Boston Studies in the Philosophy of Science,* vol 4. Springer. https://doi.org/10.1007/978-94-010-3378-7_2.

World Health Organisation (WHO). (2001). *International Classification of Functioning, Disability and Health.* WHO.

Zhang, P., Duan, L., Ou, Y., Ling, Q., Cao, L., Qian, H., Zhang, J., Wang, J., & Yuan, X. (2023).The cerebellum and cognitive neural networks. *Frontiers in Human Neuroscience,* 17: 1197459. doi: 10.3389/fnhum.2023.1197459.

FURTHER READING

Ellis, A., & Young, A. (1988). *Human Cognitive Neuropsychology: A Textbook with Readings.* Psychology Press; Taylor & Francis.

Felson Duchan, J., & Byng, S. (Eds.). (2004). *Challenging Aphasia Therapies: Broadening the Discourse and Extending the Boundaries.* Psychology Press; Taylor & Francis.

Hillis, A. E. (Ed.). (2015). *The Handbook of Adult Language Disorders,* 2nd ed. Psychology Press.

LPAA Project Group. (2001). Life participation approach to aphasia: a statement of values for the future. In R. Chapey (Ed.), *Language Intervention Strategies in Aphasia and Related Neurogenic Communication Disorders*, 4th ed. (pp. 235–245). Lippincott, Williams & Wilkins.

Martin, N., Thompson, C. K., & Worrall, L. (2008). *Aphasia Rehabilitation: The Impairment and Its Consequences*. Plural Publishing.

Papathanasiou, Ilias & Coppens, Patrick (2022). *Aphasia and Related Neurogenic Communication Disorders*. 3rd ed. Jones and Bartlett Learning.

Parr, S., Pound, C., Byng, S., & Moss, B. (2004). *The Stroke and Aphasia Handbook*. Connect Press.

Pound, C., Parr, S., Lindsay, J., & Woolf, C. (2000). *Beyond Aphasia: Therapies for Living with Communication Disability*. Speechmark Winslow Press.

Rapp, B. (Ed.) (2002). *The Handbook of Cognitive Neuropsychology. What Deficits Reveal about the Human Mind*. Psychology Press. https://doi.org/10.4324/9781315783017

Simmons-Mackie, N., King Fischer, J., & Beukelman, D. R. (2013). *Supporting Communication for Adults with Acute and Chronic Aphasia*. Brookes Publishing.

Chapter 3

APHASIA MANAGEMENT

18 BEST PRACTICE

Management involves having an overview of the key areas your client needs you to provide input for, such as assessment, goal setting, outcome measures, return to work, ending therapy. Your management should follow relevant **clinical guidelines** (see Appendix 5), how the service where you work operates and best practice recommendations for working with people with aphasia (see the Aphasia United Best Practice Recommendations for Aphasia in Appendix 3). Your management of an individual client starts with understanding their relevant **medical issues** and the causes of their aphasia, and an **understanding of recovery** from aphasia. Most people experience some recovery, and it involves spontaneous recovery, neural plasticity and therapy.

19 RECOVERY AND PROGNOSIS

In the first two weeks after a stroke, the recovery of brain activity and function occurs as a result of a reduction of the swelling in the brain, an improvement in blood flow and the subsequent repair of some damaged brain tissue. Consequently, there is usually **spontaneous recovery** of language functions, particularly speech production. In the next six months, there is further spontaneous recovery and neural reorganisation, guided by therapy, which is a longer and more complex process.

KEY FACTORS PREDICTING RECOVERY FROM APHASIA AND PROGNOSIS

Judging what potential there is for improvement and predicting recovery from aphasia is not straightforward, and various factors connect and interact, with great variation in how much improvement there is in language function and how quickly it occurs. There is evidence that, in general, recovery is influenced by factors including:

- **Lesion size:** The size of a lesion represents the degree of damage to an area of the brain. You cannot reliably estimate long-term prognosis by the severity of the brain lesion alone. The extent of the brain damage may determine the level and prognosis of aphasia at the acute stages of a stroke, but may not determine how severe it is after 12 months.
- **Location of lesions:** Acquired aphasia results from damage to the temporal, frontal and parietal regions in the left-hemisphere of the brain, which are critical for language. Damage to the arcuate fasciculus, a neural pathway connecting the parietal and temporal cortex to the frontal lobe, is key. The level of damage to this pathway has a significant impact on the severity of the aphasia and on improvements in, for example, spontaneous speech. In fact, even where the lesions are small, if the arcuate fasciculus is damaged, there is less improvement in language functions. Even a large lesion in other brain areas may have little effect on language functions. When the left superior temporal gyrus and basal ganglia are preserved there may be good recovery. See Further Reading for suggestions of where to find diagrams of the brain with sites of lesions.
- **Severity of aphasia at the onset:** How severe the aphasia is may affect prognosis; with slower and/or less improvement of language functions when someone's aphasia is initially severe. Aphasia severity after two months is strongly associated with aphasia severity after twelve months. However, after three months the degree of improvement in language functions and the severity of aphasia varies greatly, with

many people improving (Lazar et al. 2008) so that how severe someone's aphasia is at three months does not predict severity after twelve months.
- **Time since onset of the aphasia:** Time post onset does not necessarily predict how someone will respond to treatment. Recovery may not progress linearly, and there are often different recovery patterns in the first six months and the second six months.
- **Therapy:** While it is still unclear how functional reorganization happens and what language outcomes may occur, neural plasticity gives the encouragement that despite the brain lesions, there is potential for people with aphasia to improve their language and communication. Importantly, neural plasticity and recovery from aphasia depends on someone having the **appropriate type and amount of treatment** because it is the brain experiencing the behavioural therapy that brings about the making of new neural networks, heals damaged ones, teaches new strategies and recovers language function. See Chapter 9.
- **Other factors:** The aetiology of a stroke may play a part in recovery (there is some evidence that there is more recovery from aphasia caused by a haemorrhagic stroke than from an ischaemic stroke). Younger brains may have the potential for greater neural plasticity, but factors including age, sex, handedness, education and depression have **not** been found to be strong predictors of recovery. It is important for the therapist to consider an individual's personality, education history and learning abilities, level of motivation, social life and family support. These have an impact on someone's pre-existing communication habits, wishes and abilities and on the impact of the communication disorder and their relationship to therapy.

TALKING ABOUT RECOVERY AND PROGNOSIS: EDUCATION, ENCOURAGEMENT AND BALANCE

When someone with aphasia talks about recovery, explore what the word means to them. Are they looking for a return to how their speech and language was before the brain lesion or an improvement on how their communication was in the first days and weeks? You may need to clarify what has been said about recovery: people may have heard timelines and predictions from some medical staff. 'We were told that there would be no recovery after 12 months'; or 'we were told we only have a year to see any changes, after that it's too late' are reports often given to SLTs by the family of people with aphasia. Try to ensure that there is a shared understanding of what recovery means. Give information and explanations about the brain, about what has happened because of the lesion(s) and about recovery. Use drawings and diagrams. Do not assume that someone has already had the stroke or brain tumour or aphasia explained to them. Go through the relevant factors that may affect their recovery as appropriate to that person at that time. Make sure that clients and their families are aware of the potential neural plasticity gives for improvement and that they understand neurorehabilitation and the importance of therapy for recovery. Emphasise that the nature of change after a brain lesion is slow, unpredictable and variable. Take the opportunity to emphasise that what they do is key to any change, both during therapy sessions and in daily life; that their regular practice (repetition of exercises given) and learning new ways to communicate (use of strategies in conversation) is essential (see Chapter 9). Find a balance in your answers; be explicit that you cannot guarantee what improvements may occur, or what therapy will be able to achieve. And also encourage hope and engagement in therapy by telling them what evidence there is for the improvements therapy can bring for communication problems of people with aphasia. Be clear about the uncertainty. Many people with aphasia will surprise you with their recovery and change. Others with their slow or negligible recovery.

20 NEURAL PLASTICITY

The ability of the brain to reorganise its structure and connections is due to neural plasticity, which is the amazing ability of the brain to recover its functions following damage.

Neuro-imaging studies (e.g. MRI and fMRI) show the structural and functional changes that can take place. The brain can use undamaged parts of the brain to take over the tasks that damaged parts used to carry out. It is not known which areas of the brain are involved, although, in principle, language function can be supported by areas of the brain other than the established left-hemisphere language network (see PLORAS in Further Reading). The possibilities are:

- Repair of damaged areas, with a return to function of core left-hemisphere language regions
- Redistribution of functions to healthy parts of the brain: perhaps neural networks in the brain tissue around the lesion are reconstructed, or the surviving brain regions reorganise cerebral connections so they can take on new or expanded roles in language processing
- Involvement of the opposite hemisphere, which takes over the functions of the damaged hemisphere.

21 GOAL SETTING

Goals can be seen as the intended outcomes of specific interventions to improve or maintain someone's communication skills. They also form a contract between the therapist and client. They should be negotiated and reviewed regularly, as they can change over time. Discuss goals with the client and their family at the first appointment and make the process collaborative. Remember that not everyone is used to thinking about 'goals' in the way we might mean and check that there is a shared understanding of goals and plans. Find out what is concerning them and why they have come for therapy. Focus on the impact of the aphasia on their everyday life. Some people with aphasia have enough speech, or other means of communicating, to discuss goals. Some have communication and/or cognitive difficulties which prevent them from understanding the language used in the conversation and/or giving much information about their hopes and goals. Supported conversation and offering alternative written/pictorial options can help here (see Chapter 10). Others have psychological difficulties such as low mood or anxiety or are still reeling from the impact of the stroke or diagnosis and may need help to focus on goal setting.

Even with support in conversation to understand and communicate wishes, the goals may only be general, perhaps, 'to get my speech back'. Bear in mind what people with aphasia usually want (Worrall et al. 2011), this may be: a return to their life before the aphasia – to their work, social and leisure activities and to be able to communicate (not only basic needs but also their thoughts and opinions). These are goals that link to the *ICF* (e.g. Activities and Participation) and this framework can be used in sessions to discuss goals (see WHO 2001).

Someone's long-term goal might be to find the words they want to say in everyday conversation, independently, to return to their previous social life. This goal points to looking at their word retrieval and sentence processing difficulties, their ability to manage group conversations, what strategies and support can improve their participation in conversations. Your initial observations will suggest appropriate assessments to understand these better (see Chapter 4). The therapy plan emerges from the information that the goal setting and assessment gives you. Use the long-term goals that have been agreed, and divide them into clear, smaller goals or targets. Make it clear that the therapy suggested aims to reach the long-term goals. For example, a broad goal might be to make phone calls. This could include smaller goals such as working on spoken word production which may need semantic and/or phonological therapy; use of strategies such as circumlocution, written word list; practice in sessions with the therapist; support from family to motivate, provide reminders and back-up while making the phone call.

Make sure everyone understands the goals agreed. Be clear how assessment and therapy fit into the goals and what each person's role is in working towards them. This makes it more likely that the client engages with therapy, both in and outside sessions, because the tasks relate directly and clearly to their wishes.

At the first appointment, KW explained, using fluent spontaneous speech in conversation, that she was having word finding difficulties (WFD). These were making her lose confidence in her ability to continue teaching and she was fearful of losing her job. She explained that her main concern was to keep working, and she was looking to therapy to help her achieve that goal.

An assessment of word finding put her in a normal range in terms of raw scores; she was able to access the correct form of the target word, but the extra time it took her to name items or find words in conversation was also measured and noted as having a significant impact on the pre-stroke speed and fluency of her speech. She knew that the reduction in fluency and the hesitations in her speech were noticed by others and this was having an impact on how her everyday conversations were going and on her confidence.

Aphasia therapy for KW involved education about aphasia and word retrieval errors, strategies to manage these (including educating her family and friends about aphasia, word finding difficulties and how to help KW in conversation) and targeted practice of relevant words.

KW said that the information about aphasia, learning what word retrieval difficulties were and the reason for the hesitations in her speech in conversation made the changes in her speech less bewildering. One goal was to manage the WFD as they happened, so therapy included developing strategies for this; suggesting different options for KW to trial and choose. Family and friends were asked to help in different ways; particularly to give KW time and space and patience and to continue to engage with her in conversations as they always had. Therapy also involved repetition of lists of words relevant to her work.

Management and therapy points: KW could easily have been discharged at the assessment if the raw scores on the assessment sheets were the only thing looked at;

> it was important to note (and measure) the impact of the delay in accessing words, to listen to her concerns and to her experience of the impact of the aphasia on her activities (her work) and participation (in conversation), and therapy prioritised her goal to maintain her job; which she did.

22 MOTIVATION

It is important that a client is motivated in therapy, and this is helped by ensuring that they are an active participant and that the goals for therapy are chosen by the client, clearly agreed and obviously related to the therapy tasks in sessions. Motivation can be difficult in the face of being told that there are no guarantees of improvement, while also being asked to put a lot of effort and time in to the therapy and practice. Make sure that your client is sufficiently aware of the nature of aphasia, of what 'getting better' can mean. Therapy should include improving self-monitoring, so that your client develops their ability to use and adapt strategies and to recognise successes as well as errors.

This is important for motivation; be careful not to focus solely on what is wrong with a client's communication; make sure that from the first time you meet them you also talk about success: ask about 'good' conversations; encouraging everyone to see these as times when there was success in getting a message across. 'When did you understand what he was trying to say, and how?' This is also the start of working on improving self-monitoring and total communication strategies (see Point 82). Point out that successful communication can include words that are not accurate, partly correct or errors. Part of the education about aphasia is that the number of these errors will vary from day to day, within a day and even within a conversation because that is the nature of aphasia. Remind the client that it is common to be hyper-aware of errors and to not notice the success in conversation. Note whether the person with aphasia and their conversation partner tend to meet errors with negative responses. There are clients who respond to errors with self-sabotaging remarks such as, 'I'm terrible' or 'I'm useless'. Part of therapy is to help them accept errors and to focus on the wider issue of being understood, acknowledging and/or encouraging them to keep trying to communicate, despite the errors, reminding them that success is about getting their message across and worth noting, as well as the number of errors made.

You will be working with someone's pre-existing personality and attitude towards change, disability, what is acceptable, what is possible. Although we read about people with tremendous drive following adversity, we should not expect everyone to have that approach. Group therapy provides an opportunity for people to hear different responses to illness and aphasia. There is usually a range of responses, but some people will voice a commitment to their goals and some self-confidence, even in the face of a continuing effort to work towards something which may not be attainable, with the understanding that if they give up, they definitely won't attain it. You will also realise that without motivation on the part of the person with aphasia, you can offer therapy, but they may not want it or be ready for it.

23 RETURN TO WORK

Even in the early days of their aphasia, many people think about getting back to work. You may consider this unrealistic, that they are in denial about the extent and impact of their communication difficulties. It can be tempting to brush the questions about work aside, to be non-committal or even hope that you can avoid the subject altogether. But it is important to remember that it makes sense for people with aphasia and their families to be thinking of going back to work; it is not only important for economic and social reasons, but, for most people, work is a key part of their life, important for self-esteem. Being back at work is also symbolic of being 'better', back to 'normal'. So, you should expect the topic to come up and goal setting should include looking at a return to work.

Relate goals to potential work demands and find out what is needed to help a return to work. It can be a useful exercise to suggest that the person with aphasia and their partner talk about and make a written list of the actions, activities and tasks they did at work. You can suggest that they imagine being at work for a day and go through in detail what they are doing; include the journey there, what will they be expected to do? In that way they start to make the idea of being back at work more concrete and they may see that while some of the activities are still accessible for them, others are too demanding and would need to be changed/revised/removed. Sometimes by talking through a typical day at work with their partner, and then with you, the reality of the demands of their work sinks in. Therapy goals can be built around the demands identified, and include working on understanding and using specific, work-related words. Preparing to return to work usually needs careful and detailed planning, across disciplines including occupational therapy and occupational health. Some people may need to find college courses to develop skills and knowledge.

> Peter was in his mid-twenties when he sustained an ABI as a result of a car accident. He made a good recovery in terms of his ability to communicate. Goal planning included return to work planning, analysing what his work involved and demanded from him in terms of language and cognitive skills. He identified concentration, language processing (reading, technical conversations) as key. He arranged a gradual return to work to manage his fatigue which had a significant impact on his language and cognitive skills. He was very concerned about having to repeat the story of what had happened to him, so an important part of his SLT was to plan and practise a 'speech' to his colleagues. He worked on writing

> a narrative and rehearsing it in therapy sessions and answering possible questions. He went back to work, prepared to present himself to his old team.

What would constitute a 'return to work' and a successful outcome for someone? Does going back to work mean going back to the same job or can someone be flexible about possible changes to their work (perhaps to a different position which is at a lower grade, with lower pay, in the same company). Would this be a more realistic option than getting a new job in a new company? Would they consider voluntary work rather than paid work? How much therapy would be needed and for how long to rebuild the skills needed? Can you predict whether targeted therapy would bring about the changes needed to mean that this client could be back doing some or all of their previous role?

> Henry was a founding director of a successful company. His conversational speech was effective, and he was a good communicator, using whatever speech he had confidently and adding appropriate gestures, facial expressions and involving his listener in facilitating the conversation. His personality and his understanding that communication goes beyond speech meant that, despite the occasional word errors and word retrieval difficulties, he would usually get his message across in a conversation. He managed well at work in a new role that took him into another area of the company. However, his aphasia included dyscalculia (difficulties processing numbers and calculations), and auditory processing difficulties which made following group conversations difficult. Therapy improved his auditory processing significantly, so that he could understand more in both one-to-one and group

> conversations. He improved his ability to manage numbers, but still needed support to understand and use them reliably. He was 'let go' by the company. He had time to come to terms with the change in his life and while sad, was positive about the end of his working life.

Communication difficulties continue to be more of a barrier to acceptance (see Chapter 10). Sadly, many people with aphasia do lose their job and it is often the aphasia, rather than physical disabilities, that prevent the return to work or mean that someone is unable to continue in a role. Of course, it depends on how willing their employer is to make any useful adjustments to their work (e.g. workload, extra support, allowing for gradual return to work, reduced hours) and the type of work they are going back to (how much speaking, writing, reading, listening, use of numbers/calculations they are required to do). Sometimes larger companies are more able to provide support for a successful return.

> Margaret had a job with a utility firm and following her stroke, her aphasia meant that she had very limited speech and limited writing, with good auditory comprehension and reading and good use of numbers and calculations. She was still able to work from home on her computer doing the spreadsheets. She was pleased that her work had kept her on, it was financially important, but the work she was now doing was only part of her role prior to her stroke and she missed the conversations and camaraderie of work. After a few months, the firm needed someone who could take part in the meetings and discussions, and she was one of the people 'let go' in a round of redundancies. This was a blow to Margaret, both financially and emotionally.

24 ENDING THERAPY (DISCHARGE)

Begin the discussion about discharge when talking about goals and treatment options; frame the therapy process as having a beginning and an end. It can be overwhelming for some people to think about discharge, but an important goal of any therapy is to manage the inevitable end of treatment. This may be because your health service has made decisions about what it will provide. There will be financial constraints on your SLT service. Your client's health insurance policy will have limits on what it will cover, and individuals will have a budget or limit that they can afford to pay for therapy. Make sure that if you have six sessions to offer, you are open about why this is. Do not suggest that this is all the input someone necessarily needs or would benefit from.

Reviewing goals can be helpful when you consider discharge. Discharging someone may seem appropriate because they are not achieving their goals but consider whether improvements may still be possible if goals were more sensitive, and therapy refocused. Decisions to discharge someone with PPA, when deterioration in communication skills is inevitable, needs careful discussion and goal setting.

25 MEASURING OUTCOMES

Measuring outcomes of therapy is part of professional practice. Remember to take baseline measurements before starting therapy input, after therapy and, if you can, take them three, six and twelve months later too. We need to evaluate our therapy, using clinical assessments and outcome measures to evaluate the progress and outcomes of therapy intervention and its impact on someone's goals. Outcome measurements enable us to check that the therapy we have been doing is having the desired effect on the language impairments and functional language skills of a person with aphasia, and to change interventions where necessary. You could use the Scenario Test (Swinburn, Porter & Howard 2023) to measure multimodal communication. Measure impairment (e.g. the Comprehensive

Aphasia Test (CAT)); function observations made by someone's spouse or partner can provide another measure of a client's functional communication, e.g. the Communication Effectiveness Index (CETI)(Lomas et al. 1989); goal (Goal Attainment Scale), self-reported measurements of mood (e.g. Stroke Aphasia Depression Scale – The Stroke and Aphasia Quality Of Life Scale-39 (SAQOL) (Hilari & Byng 2001); Depression Intensity Scale Circles (DISCs) (Turner-Stokes et al. 2005); quality of life (e.g. Adult Carer QOL questionnaire (Ac-QOL) (Elwick et al. 2010)). The CAT can be used to measure outcomes of treatment on the language impairments. Often SLT services need to justify their value, and showing the improvements in standardised outcome measures can be one way of doing this. There are validated outcome measurement tools, e.g. the Therapy Outcome Measure (TOM) (Enderby & John 2020), a clinician-reported measure which is simple to use and describes a client's strengths and weaknesses in the areas of impairment, activity, participation and well-being. Measures can be taken when someone is first seen and on discharge from therapy. Asking the person with aphasia to report/comment on outcomes can be done via measures such as the Aphasia Impact Questionnaire which is part of the CAT and supports the subjective rating of the impact of the aphasia on everyday life. This can also be a useful way of beginning to look at goal setting. The POWERS (see Further Reading) analyses whether word finding improves after a period of therapy, measuring word production in natural conversation. Another useful way of discussing goals and outcomes is to use the A-FROM, another guide to outcome measurement in aphasia. This looks at impairment, personal identity, environment and participation; all important areas to measure the outcomes of aphasia therapy intervention (Kagan 1998) (see Appendix 1 for the model). The Aphasia Institute (https://www.aphasia.ca) also offers the Basic Outcome Measure Protocol for Aphasia (BOMPA), which uses supported conversation to assess aphasia severity, participation in conversation and quality of life.

26 PRESSURES ON MANAGEMENT

Clinical guidelines may set out a level of therapy you should provide, but there are significant pressures on SLTs to manage their aphasia caseload. In acute hospitals, the service is often required to focus on dysphagia (swallowing problems), and this reduces time spent on communication (Foster et al. 2014). It can be difficult for therapists whose interest is in working with people with aphasia and whose job has a mixed caseload because they see the aphasia work 'swallowed up' by this focus on dysphagia. Look to other aphasia clinicians to support your work; discuss ways to balance the focus on dysphagia with the communication needs of clients; some clinicians have aimed to provide informal communication assessments during dysphagia sessions. Join aphasia clinical excellence networks (CENs) and the British Aphasiology Society. Look both nationally and internationally for resources (see Appendix 5 Useful Resources).

27 BRAIN TUMOUR

The management of someone's aphasia when they have a brain tumour will have some differences from that of someone after a stroke or TBI. Aphasia occurs in around 30– 50 per cent of people with a left-hemisphere brain tumour resection. At the acute recovery stage, the aphasia you will see may be very different from people who have had a stroke; often there are only mild word retrieval difficulties, regardless of the location of the lesion or the tumour grade. Because the difficulties are so different from post-stroke aphasia and can be mild, they are often undetected and overlooked. Part of our management is to make sure that all health-care staff are aware of the aphasia and of how to support communication at all stages of care. At the chronic stage, the choice of assessment is important (CAT findings are possibly the most reliable) (Brownsett et al. 2019). Therapy promotes the use of different strategies in conversation. Brain tumours are the biggest cancer killer of people under 40 so you may be working with someone younger than many of your clients over a shorter time, perhaps more intensively. Your management of goal setting may include supporting conversations about someone's wishes for end-of-life care.

28 MANAGEMENT AT ACUTE STAGE

The **acute stage** of aphasia recovery after a stroke refers to the initial 4–6 weeks, the **subacute stage** to the next 12 months. The **chronic stage** of recovery follows this and can last for several years. **Management at the acute stage** involves assessment to diagnose the communication problems; implementing a therapy programme; education about aphasia (for the person with aphasia, family and health/care staff); counselling and advocacy (Foster et al. 2014). Many SLTs working in the acute sector report there are **barriers** to carrying out assessment and therapy. This is despite the significant, negative impact that having a communication impairment has on people who are on a hospital ward. They are less satisfied with the general health care they receive and have poorer outcomes in health and rehabilitation. Often, the provision of SLT services to people with aphasia in the acute hospital is inconsistent with best-practice recommendations because, despite clinical guidelines, the pressures of the high number of people to treat on the ward by a relatively small number of clinicians, an uncertainty about what therapy to provide and an increased focus on dysphagia management all limit the amount and quality of the provision of aphasia therapy.

ASSESSMENT (SEE CHAPTER 4 AND APPENDIX 4)

Early assessment is important and there are standardised assessments aimed at the acute setting, which are relatively quick and easy to administer. Many services also develop their own screening tests or non-standardised assessments for use on the ward, with a focus on informal conversations and observations. It can be difficult for someone with aphasia at the acute stage to cooperate with screening or assessment, due to medical factors alongside the aphasia, including: fatigue, confusion, distress, anxiety, cognitive difficulties and a lack of motivation to try and communicate. The assessments carried out by other professionals on the hospital ward (occupational therapists, neuropsychologists, clinical psychologists, nurses) can inform your understanding of someone's reactions to your assessments. You will need to be flexible and return to see someone to carry out whatever small bits of assessment are possible, bearing in mind the importance of aphasia assessment: a lack of response to verbal questions and/or speech which is poor in content can be mistaken for confusion, for example, by other professionals. Your assessment is essential to differentiate these. Your supportive assessment can reveal language abilities and competence. Your assessment looks for ways that someone can better understand information by presenting it in different modalities and reducing the linguistic complexity. By supporting communication, you may find that someone with significant comprehension difficulties can be enabled to understand better and indicate choices. Sharing this information is part of your role as advocate (also see Point 69).

The assessment you do in the acute stage will reflect someone's abilities at that time but is likely to change rapidly, requiring monitoring and further assessment. In terms of what assessment tells us about **diagnosis** and **prognosis**, in the acute setting you are working with an evolving situation; the spontaneous recovery that occurs (see Point 19) leads to changes in the ways the aphasia presents in individual clients in the early days, weeks and months. Someone who initially has no speech production at all may regain some speech and then present with e.g. word retrieval difficulties.

GOAL SETTING

At the acute stage, the discussion around goals may initially be with family and staff as much as with the person with aphasia. Goals may focus on activities and participation on the ward with the communication demands of everyday tasks such as eating and washing. Goals for communication could include using communication charts with medical staff and family; establishing a consistent way of indicating yes or no; a further, wider goal to ensure that supported conversation is used by everyone on the ward who engages with the person with aphasia.

THERAPY IN THE ACUTE AND SUBACUTE STAGES

When working with someone with aphasia at these stages it may seem that they are only 'passing through'; waiting to be discharged or transferred. Not on the ward long enough for therapy, or not well enough to engage. However, while it is unclear whether people gain from starting therapy in the first two weeks rather than after four weeks, the first three months after a stroke is a critical time for brain recovery and rehabilitation. Therapy that starts within the first month can achieve greater gains than when it starts in the chronic recovery stage (Godecke et al. 2014).

WHAT SORT OF THERAPY

While it may be best practice for treatment of aphasia to be given at the acute and subacute stages as well as chronic stage of recovery, there are no standardised levels or recommended types of treatment at the acute or subacute stages of aphasia. There is growing evidence of what type of therapy (and how much) is useful to guide interventions in these first few months that can bring positive change to language processing, including cognitive-linguistic interventions (e.g. semantic feature therapy, cued naming therapy). The Very Early Rehabilitation in SpEech (VERSE) trial (Godecke et al. 2021) used therapy tasks such as single word picture naming, sentence level practice with picture description.

HOW MUCH THERAPY

Look at best practice recommendations such as the *NICE Clinical Guidelines* (NICE 2023) to guide management. There is evidence that daily aphasia therapy can improve the communication outcomes in people with both moderate and severe aphasia in the very early stage of recovery from a stroke. Recruited between 0–10 days post stroke, people received daily impairment-based therapy for between 30 and 80 minutes while in hospital (Godecke et al. 2012) (see Appendix 5). Someone's ability to communicate effectively can improve despite their moderate or severe aphasia if they have daily therapy when on the acute ward. Alongside initiating impairment-based therapy, other input is vital at the acute and subacute stages, such as **total communication** and **supported conversation** (see Point 82). Once you know what someone's speech and language difficulties and remaining skills are, therapy can include establishing and practising using helpful strategies to help someone understand others and get their message across. Strategies may be using writing and/or gestures alongside or instead of speech; augmentative and alternative communication (AAC) from simple communication charts, where there are pictures and/or words to point to, to more complex apps (see Point 81).

EDUCATION

Promoting better communication in everyday situations involves educating and informing staff on the ward, family and friends about how to communicate with the person with aphasia. It should both cover the essential information about what aphasia is and be specific to the individual. Everyone who engages with someone with aphasia should know that they need to find out how that person may indicate a yes or no response more reliably, using gesture or pointing, for example. This includes health care assistants who offer food and drink on the ward. Make sure that if someone has a communication chart that everyone on the ward knows how to use it and try and monitor that it is used. Make it relevant to the person with aphasia; it might be that they can only manage two or three pictures on the communication chart at once. Or that using written words instead of/alongside speech when they ask questions helps comprehension. Make sure that the information about someone's aphasia is highlighted and shared by all; this **advocacy** for communication is an essential part of your role at every stage. You may deliver training in communicating with people with aphasia to the multidisciplinary team (MDT) on the ward. This is often given in the form of **supported communication partner** training for family and staff. The education about aphasia you give people with aphasia and their families at the acute stage becomes a form of counselling (see Chapter 10).

> 'They've been giving him coffee to drink, and he hasn't drunk it because he hates coffee!'
>
> 'I couldn't even say yes or no to anyone about sugar in my tea.'
>
> 'No one spoke to me.'
>
> These reports are from family and from people with aphasia who initially had no speech on the ward and were not provided with another way to get their message across.

Beyond the one-to-one SLT input, the environment of an acute ward is important for aphasia recovery. Following a stroke, in the first weeks as an inpatient, people with aphasia commonly spend less than 30 per cent of their day communicating. This lack of communication not only inhibits any recovery of language skills, but there is a risk of developing a new habit of not using speech or language, which can have a negative impact on someone's ability to engage with rehabilitation. Could hospital wards become environments that promote more use of language, with less time alone and silent and more social and cognitive activity? Education about aphasia, training in supporting conversation can help promote more communication on the ward. Of course, how possible it is to create these environments depends on the ward, on how many staff are available, on time pressures as well as how physically well and able to engage the person with aphasia is. Wherever you can, try to champion the communication needs of people with aphasia in the acute and subacute settings.

ADDRESSING DISCHARGE

Keep detailed records of assessments, including speech samples; if you add to joint notes on the ward, make sure you have written information to pass on to your colleagues in community services on discharge. Look at what can be done if someone is discharged from the hospital but has a long wait for further SLT input in the community. Make sure the family has details of the onward referral process and how to access more SLT, either via the NHS or an independent therapist. There is potential for improvement with therapy at the early subacute stage, so make sure that you provide therapy practice to be continued at home, along with the information about aphasia.

29 ABI

At the acute and subacute stage you may see aphasia in only 1–2.5 per cent of people following an ABI, although it has been reported as high as 32 per cent. After an ABI, 75–100 per cent of people have cognitive-communication disorders and cognitive abilities such as attention and initiation have a significant impact on communication abilities (see Chapter 5). As when working with people after a stroke, many SLTs find that they face significant barriers working with people with communication difficulties after an ABI at the acute stage. These include time constraints and size of caseload, making a thorough initial communication assessment difficult. The responsibilities for speaking valve placement, dysphagia and tracheostomy, for example, can take priority over cognitive-communication concerns at the acute stage. There is usually more time available for communication therapy at the subacute and chronic stages, often on neurorehabilitation units.

30 MANAGEMENT OF CHRONIC APHASIA

Around 31 per cent of people after their first stroke will have aphasia at the acute stage and 50–60 per cent of these people will still have it 12 months later. People with chronic post-stroke aphasia (e.g. after five years) can continue to improve. At what point improvements occur varies, depending on the aphasia and the therapy given. There is good evidence to expect and pursue improvement, even when prognosis is uncertain. The difficulty for many SLT services in the NHS in the UK is that there is a lack of funding for a service to provide adequate amounts of therapy to people with chronic aphasia. This means there is often a lack of service provision for people with aphasia rather than a lack of potential in people with aphasia to improve (see Chapter 9 for more on chronic aphasia).

31 MANAGEMENT OF PROGRESSIVE APHASIA

Dementia involves significant, progressive damage to brain cells leading to a loss of cognitive function, including memory and language. The most common cause is Alzheimer's (AD) where amyloid plaques and tau tangles gradually accumulate in the brain; these disrupt neuron function resulting in cell death. Vascular dementia (VaD) results from cerebrovascular disease, vascular conditions/heart disease that led to vascular lesions in the brain with an abrupt onset in cognitive function and a progression of symptoms in small stages. Neurodegenerative disorders include dementia with Lewy bodies (DLB) and Parkinson's disease with dementia, with cognitive impairments alongside the extrapyramidal symptoms. There is also mixed dementia (with features of AD and VaD or features of AD and DLB).

FRONTOTEMPORAL LOBAR DEGENERATION (FTD/FTLD) AND PROGRESSIVE APHASIAS

FTD disorders or primary progressive aphasias (PPAs) are the result of degeneration of the frontal and temporal lobes of the brain with loss of function. It is less common than aphasia after stroke, but you are likely to have some clients with PPA during your career as an aphasia therapist. There are different types of PPA: **progressive non-fluent aphasia (PNFA)**, also known as non-fluent variant PPA (**nfvPPA**), speech is hesitant and effortful due to difficulties with single word retrieval and with sentence production. There are also reading, writing and calculation difficulties. Use of gestures may also deteriorate. Language comprehension is relatively preserved, at least in the early stages of the disease. **PPA – semantic (PPA-S)** or **semantic variant PPA (svPPA)** describes difficulties seen with word comprehension and naming that can progress to **semantic dementia (SD)**, involving a profound loss of semantic knowledge, with poor understanding of words, and semantic errors in speech. Speech is fluent and grammatically correct. Cognitive functions that do not depend on meaning are well preserved. **Logopenic progressive aphasia (PPA-L or LPA or lvPPA)** communication involves slow and hesitant speech caused by word retrieval difficulties (sentence production remains good). There is good single word comprehension initially, but comprehension of longer sentences or linguistically more complex information becomes steadily more difficult. There is also **PPA +** (when there are other cognitive deficits alongside aphasia) and **PPA extended** (when the language symptoms of another PPA subtype also develop).

SLT MANAGEMENT OF PPA

There are key differences from the aphasia you see after a stroke; it is often unclear what the diagnosis is, or how long someone has been having difficulties with communication. There will be significant cognitive deficits to assess or understand. Your work is in the context of an inevitable decline in abilities, but people with PPA generally live for several years following diagnosis, and their language difficulties and needs change over time. You will benefit from clinical discussions with other SLTs working with these clients. As well as the traditional aphasia therapist role of helping someone to manage the changes in language functions and promote the best conversations possible, your roles may include helping to **diagnose** which type of PPA someone has, **monitoring** someone's communication decline or progression of the disease to inform the MDT as well as family and **optimising** communication for as long as possible. **Goals** need to be flexible and revisited frequently to be relevant and appropriate and to make sure that any treatment is meeting the client's changing needs. **Assessment in PPA** screening and assessing someone's speech and language skills and the impact of the cognitive deficits on communication (using informal, formal assessment; see Chapter 4) contributes to the clinical management of people with dementia; both your SLT input and that of the MDT. PPAs present as complex disorders and are often difficult to diagnose.

THERAPY

With the focus on continuing to participate in daily activities, therapy will aim to preserve any and all language functions and better conversations (see Chapters 9 and 10). **Impairment-based** therapy for single word naming and using script or narrative writing at sentence level has been shown to enable people with PPA to maintain function and even to make improvements in word retrieval and speech fluency. Therapies can involve practising personalised and functionally useful lists of words (via repetition, reading aloud, writing). This therapy may be most successful earlier in the course of the disease, so it is important to be pro-active and start therapy early. VNeST therapy (Edmonds, Nadeau & Kiran 2009) may be a preventative treatment for word retrieval skills, preserving the semantic links between words. Improvement in word retrieval treatments can last for 6–12 months. Generalisation is variable and can depend on PPA subtype (better for lvPPA and nfvPPA than for svPPA). As with all aphasia therapy, it is vital for people to do the home practice. Cognitive changes for these clients include apathy so watch for a loss of motivation to carry out the practice. **Communication support, strategies, AAC.** As with the impairment-based therapy, introduce total communication strategies early in therapy to make them more acceptable and more likely to be used. (See Chapter 9, Point 81). As someone's disease progresses, it may be appropriate to substitute the impairment-based lexical retrieval therapy with more practice of strategies, using drawing and/or gesture in conversation. This work has to involve training the people living and/or working with someone with PPA to be communication partners. This communication skills training is very much what we would do with the family of someone with aphasia after a stroke; aiming to encourage strategies that can enable communication (e.g. gesture) and reducing those aspects of conversation that can make communication more difficult, such as giving too much information at once and interrupting. Better Conversations with Aphasia is a resource created for people with aphasia after stroke and the principles have been used to create Better Conversations with PPA (BCPPA) (see Further Reading and Chapter 10). Key to SLT input is **supporting family, friends and carers** to maintain the best conversation possible for as long as possible. Remember that information and peer support can help to provide important psychological support as well as practical advice about navigating this complex disease and maintaining communication for as long as possible (see Chapter 10 and Further Reading below). As well as the one-to-one support, give information in appropriate handouts, group therapy where possible, information about how to access group therapy and/or a lay support group where these are available if your service does not offer this.

32 BILINGUAL FACTORS

Management is stipulated by clinical guidelines (e.g. *National Clinical Guidelines for Stroke*, NICE 2023) including the use of interpreters for assessment and provision of information, therapy and practice in the preferred language.

There are some standardised assessments translated into other languages (see Appendix 4). Find out during assessment which language your client usually speaks, reads and writes. In 2021, 91.1 per cent of the population in England had English as a main language.[1] If there is another language used, you will need to know which language(s) and which is first acquired and/or most used. In 2021, the most common other languages in England and Wales were: Polish (1.1 per cent), Romanian (0.8 per cent), Panjabi (0.5 per cent) and Urdu (0.5 per cent). These are small numbers of people relative to the population, but your individual caseload may contain higher percentages of bilingual clients, depending on where you work.

It is important to be aware of the pre-stroke language proficiencies of a bilingual client. Find out what level of English was understood and used prior to the aphasia, which languages are routinely spoken at home and which languages are spoken by everyone in the family. You will need to be aware of the abilities of the family members to understand and use English; and how much support they need to understand the information given to them about aphasia, about therapy, about supported conversation. Do you have access to information about aphasia in the languages of those communities?

INTERPRETERS

The SLT who does not know the client's stronger, primary language will need to find either an SLT who is bilingual in both English and the language spoken by your client and/or family or an interpreter who will help carry out an assessment and discuss the findings in both languages. The strengths and weaknesses in both languages can then be discussed and treatment options explored. There is not much evidence about the provision or the success of assessment and therapy for aphasia that is delivered in a language other than English via an interpreter; this is an area that needs more research, including resources that are accessible for people with aphasia for whom English is a second language (ESL) (Larkman et al. 2022). Working with clients who are ESL or bilingual/multilingual is clinically challenging for SLTs (Centeno, Swathi & Armstrong 2020). You will need to factor in extra time for pre- and post-assessment discussions with the interpreter, including providing the interpreter with information about aphasia and about the assessments to be used. Make sure that the interpreter understands that it is important that they do not answer for the client or help the client answer, especially when there are formal assessments being done. It will also be important that they give you verbatim reports of what the client attempts to say, and that they note the errors made in speech and/or writing. It is useful to record the sessions. You will need the interpreter to help you build up any pattern of errors there may be by identifying and providing you with the incorrect words, sound errors in words and sentence errors of the client (Kong 2016). If you are able to have an interpreter for therapy as well as assessment, you will also need to train them in supported conversation strategies. It is useful to remember that some bilingual people with aphasia mix languages, even within one phrase. This can be useful for day-to-day communication (Hameau, Dmowski & Nickels 2023).

Prior to his stroke and aphasia, Mr. P was bilingual and a fluent English speaker. However, his wife could speak, but not read or write in English. Assessment had shown that Mr. P benefited from using written information and attempting writing to communicate, so working on total communication strategies and supported conversation was an agreed goal of therapy. The usual involvement of family in the therapy sessions and the home practice/conversations needed to be adjusted; in this case finding other family members who could read and write English to do the work at home with Mr. P. This was not ideal as writing was an important strategy for Mr. P and Mrs. P. could not benefit from him using it, so conversations continued to be more difficult than they might have been between them. The question of Mrs. P. attending English literacy classes was raised as something to support Mr. P in his aphasia therapy.

NOTE

1 Office for National Statistics (ONS), released 29 November 2022, ONS website, statistical bulletin, Language, England and Wales: Census 2021.

REFERENCES

Brownsett, S. L. E., Ramajoo, K., Copland, D., McMahon, K. L., Robinson, G., Drummond, K., Jeffree, R. L., Olson, S., Ong, B., & De Zubicaray, G. (2019) Language deficits following dominant hemisphere tumour resection are significantly underestimated by syndrome-based aphasia assessments. *Aphasiology*, 33(10): 1163–1181. doi: 10.1080/02687038.2019.1614760

Centeno, J., Swathi, K., & Armstrong, E. (2020). Aphasia management in growing multiethnic populations. *Aphasiology*, 34(11): 1314–1318. doi: 10.1080/02687038.2020.1781420

Edmonds, L. A., Nadeau, S. E., & Kiran, S. (2009). Effect of Verb Network Strengthening Treatment (VNeST) on lexical retrieval of content words in sentences in persons with aphasia. *Aphasiology*, 23(3): 402–424. doi: 10.1080/02687030802291339

Elwick, H., Joseph, S., Becker, S., & Becker, F. (2010). *Manual for the Adult Carer Quality of Life Questionnaire (AC-QoL)*. The Princess Royal Trust for Carers.

Enderby, P., & John, A. (Eds.). (2020). *Therapy Outcome Measure Theoretical Underpinning and Case Studies*. J & R Press.

Foster, A., O'Halloran, R., Rose, M., & Worrall, L. (2014). "Commmunic3ation is taking a back seat": speech pathologists' perceptions of aphasia management in acute hospital settings. *Aphasiology*, 30(5): 585–608. https://doi.org/10.1080/02687038.2014.985185

Godecke, E., Ciccone, N. A., Granger, A. S., Rai, T., West, D., Cream, A., Cartwright, J., & Hankey, G. J. (2014). A comparison of aphasia therapy outcomes before and after a Very Early Rehabilitation programme following stroke. *International Journal of Language & Communication Disorders*, 49(2): 149–161. doi: 10.1111/1460-6984.12074

Godecke, E., Hird, K., Lalor, E. E., Rai, T., & Phillips, M. R. (2012). Very early poststroke aphasia therapy: a pilot randomized controlled efficacy trial. *International Journal of Stroke*, 7(8): 635–644. doi: 10.1111/j.1747-4949.2011.00631.x

RECOVERY

Hameau, S., Dmowski, U., & Nickels, L. (2023). Factors affecting cross-language activation and language mixing in bilingual aphasia: a case study. *Aphasiology*, 37(8): 1149–1172, doi: 10.1080/02687038.2022.2081960

Hilari, K. and Byng, S. (2001). Measuring quality of life in people with aphasia: the Stroke Specific Quality of Life Scale. *International Journal of Language and Communication Disorders*, 36(Suppl.): 86–91.

Kagan, A. (1998). Supported conversation for adults with aphasia: methods and resources for training conversation partners. *Aphasiology*, 12(9): 816–830. doi:10.1030/02687039808249575

Kong, A. P. H. (2016). Considerations for multilingual and culturally-diverse populations. In A. P. H. Kong (Ed.), *Analysis of Neurogenic Disordered Discourse Production: From Theory to Practice*, 1st ed. (pp. 239–285). Routledge. https://doi.org/10.4324/9781315639376

Larkman, C. S., Mellahn, K., Han, W., & Rose, M. L. (2022). Aphasia rehabilitation when speech pathologists and clients do not share the same language: a scoping review. *Aphasiology*, 37(4): 635–657. https://doi.org/10.1080/02687038.2022.2035672

Lazar, R. M., Speizer, A. E., Festa, J. R., Krakauer, J. W., Marshall, R. S. (2008). Variability in language recovery after first-time Aphasia Compendium 12 stroke. *Journal of Neurology, Neurosurgery, and Psychiatry*, 79(5): 530–534.

Lomas, J., Pickard, L., Bester, S., & Zoghaib, C. (1989). The Communication Effectiveness Index: development and psychometric evaluation of a functional communication measure for adult aphasia. *Journal of Speech and Hearing Disorders*, 54(1): 113–124.

National Institute for Health and Care Excellence (NICE) (2023). *NICE Guideline [NG236] Stroke Rehabilitation in Adults Clinical Guideline*. https://www.nice.org.uk/guidance/ng236

Swinburn, K., Porter, G., & Howard D. (2023). *The Comprehensive Aphasia Test (CAT)*, 2nd ed. Routledge.

Turner-Stokes, L., Kalmus, M., Hirani, D., Clegg, F. (2005). The Depression Intensity Scale Circles (DISCS): a first evaluation of a simple assessment tool for depression in the context of brain injury. *Journal of Neurology, Neurosurgery and Psychiatry*, 76(9): 1273–1278. doi: 10.1136/jnnp.2004.050096

World Health Organisation (WHO). (2001). *International Classification of Functioning, Disability and Health*. WHO.

Worrall, L., Sherratt, S., Rogers, P., Howe, T., Hersh, D., Ferguson, A.,& Davidson, B. (2011). What people with aphasia want: their goals according to the ICF. *Aphasiology*, 25(3): 309–322. doi: 10.1080/02687038.2010.508530

FURTHER READING

Åke, S., Hartelius, L., Jakola, A. S., & Antonsson, M. (2023). Experiences of language and communication after brain-tumour treatment: a long-term follow-up after glioma surgery. *Neuropsychological Rehabilitation*, 33(7): 1225–1261. doi: 10.1080/09602011.2022.2080720

Baker, C., Foster, A. M., D'Souza, S., Godecke, E., Shiggins, C., Lamborn, E., Lanyon, L., Kneebone, I., & Rose, M. L. (2022). Management of communication disability in the first 90 days after stroke: a scoping review. *Disability and Rehabilitation*, 44(26): 8524–8538. https://doi.org/10.1080/09638288.2021.2012843

Beeke, S., Sirman, N., Beckley, F., Maxim, J., Edwards, S., Swinburn, K., & Best, W. (2013). Better conversations with aphasia: an e-learning resource. https://extend.ucl.ac.uk

Brady, M. C., Kelly, H., Godwin, J., Enderby, P., Campbell, P.. (2016). Speech and language therapy for aphasia following stroke. *Cochrane Database of Systematic Reviews* 6June 1) Art.: CD000425. doi: https://doi.org/10.1002/14651858

Brogan, E., Ciccone, N., & Godecke, E. (2020). An exploration of aphasia therapy dosage in the first six months of stroke recovery. *Neuropsychological Rehabilitation*, 31(8): 1254–1288. https://doi.org/10.1080/09602011.2020.1776135

Brogan, E., Godecke, E., & Ciccone, N. (2020). Behind the therapy door: what is "usual care" aphasia therapy in acute stroke management? *Aphasiology*, 34(10): 1291–1313. https://doi.org/10.1080/02687038.2020.1759268

Carragher, M., Steel, G., O'Halloran, R., Torabi, T., Johnson, H., Taylor, N. F., & Rose, M. (2021). Aphasia disrupts usual care: the stroke team's perceptions of delivering healthcare to patients with aphasia. *Disability and Rehabilitation*, 43(21): 3003–3014. https://doi.org/10.1080/09638288.2020.1722264

Centeno, J., Swathi, K., & Armstrong, E. (2020). Aphasia management in growing multiethnic populations. *Aphasiology*, 34(11): 1314–1318. doi: 10.1080/02687038.2020.1781420

Clancy, L., Povey, R., & Rodham, K. (2020). "Living in a foreign country": experiences of staff-patient communication in inpatient stroke settings for people with post-stroke aphasia and those supporting them. *Disability and Rehabilitation*, 42(3): 324–334. https://doi.org/10.1080/ 09638288.2018.1497716

Coffey, B. J., Threlkeld, Z. D., Foulkes, A. S., Bodien, Y. G., & Edlow, B. L. (2021). Reemergence of the language network during recovery from severe traumatic brain injury: a pilot functional MRI study. *Brain Injury*, 35(12–13): 1552–1562. https://doi.org/10 .1080/02699052.2021.1972455

Connect & Firenza, C. (2007). *How to Volunteer: A Guide for People with Aphasia*. Connect.

Cramer, S. C. et al. (2011). Harnessing neuroplasticity for clinical applications, Brain, 134(6): 1591–1609. https://doi.org/10.1093/brain/awr039

Davie, G. L., Hutcheson, K. A., Barringer, D. A., Weinberg, J. S., & Lewin, J. S. (2009). Aphasia in patients after brain tumour resection. *Aphasiology*, 23(9): 1196–1206. doi: 10.1080/02687030802436900

Denes, Gianfranco. (2016). Neural Plasticity Across the Lifespan: How the Brain Can Change. Routledge.

D'Souza, S., Hersh, D., Godecke, E., Ciccone, N., Janssen, H., & Armstrong, E. (2022) Patients' experiences of a Communication Enhanced Environment model on an acute/slow stream rehabilitation and a rehabilitation ward following stroke: a qualitative description approach. *Disability and Rehabilitation*, 44(21): 6304–6313. https://doi.org/10.1080/09638288.2021 .1965226

Døli, H., Helland, W. A., Helland, T., Næss, H., Hofstad, H., & Specht, K. (2023). Associations between stroke severity, aphasia severity, lesion location, and lesion size in acute stroke, and aphasia severity one year post stroke. *Aphasiology*, 37(2): 307–329. doi: 10.1080/02687038.2021.2013430

Edmonds, L. A., Nadeau, S. E., & Kiran, S. (2009). Effect of Verb Network Strengthening Treatment (VNeST) on lexical retrieval of content words in sentences in persons with aphasia. *Aphasiology*, 23(3): 402–424. doi: 10.1080/02687030802291339.

Eley, E., van den Berg, M., Rose, M. L., Pierce, J. E., Foster, A., Lamborn, E., & Baker, C. (2023). The effects of cognitive-linguistic interventions to treat aphasia in the first 90 days post-stroke: a systematic review. *Aphasiology*, 38(8):1351–1376. https://doi.org/10.1080/02687038.2023.2282659

Elwick, H., Joseph, S., Becker, S., & Becker, F. (2010). *Manual for the Adult Carer Quality of Life Questionnaire (AC-QoL).* The Princess Royal Trust for Carers.

Enderby, P., & John, A. (2015). Therapy Outcomes Measures for Rehabilitation Professionals, 3rd ed. J & R Press Ltd.

Enderby, P., & John, A. (2019). *Therapy Outcome Measure User Guide.* J&R Press Ltd.

Enderby, P., & John, A. (Eds.). (2020). *Therapy Outcome Measure Theoretical Underpinning and Case Studies.* J & R Press..

Godecke, E., Armstrong, E., Rai, T., Ciccone, N., Rose, M.L., Middleton, S., Whitworth, A., Holland, A,. Ellery, F., Hankey, G.J.. Cadilhac, D. A., Bernhardt, J. (2021). A randomized control trial of intensive aphasia therapy after acute stroke: the Very Early Rehabilitation for SpEech (VERSE) study. *International Journal of Stroke*, 6(5): 556–572. doi:10.1177/1747493020961926

Graham, J. R., Pereira, S., & Teasell, R. (2011). Aphasia and return to work in younger stroke survivors. *Aphasiology*, 25(8): 952–960.

Harvey, D. Y., Parchure, S., & Hamilton, R. H. (2021). Factors predicting long-term recovery from post-stroke aphasia. *Aphasiology*, 36(11): 1351–1372. https://doi.org/10.1080/02687038.2021.1966374

Herbert, R., Best, W., Hickin, J. & Howard, D. (Eds.). (2013). *Profile of Word Errors and Retrieval in Speech (POWERS).* J and R Press.

Hersh, D. (2016). Therapy in transit: managing aphasia in the early period post stroke. *Aphasiology*, 30(5): 509–516. https://doi.org/10.1080/02687038.2015.1137555

Hersh, D., Sherratt, S., Howe, T., Worrall, L., Davidson, B., & Ferguson, A. (2012). An analysis of the "goal" in aphasia rehabilitation. *Aphasiology*, 26(8): 971–984. https://doi.org/10.1080/02687038.2012.684339

Hersh, D., Wood, P., & Armstrong, E. (2018) Informal aphasia assessment, interaction and the development of the therapeutic relationship in the early period after stroke. *Aphasiology*, 32(8): 876–901. https://doi.org/10.1080/02687038.2017.1381878

Hersh, D., Worrall, L., Banszki, F., Bennington, C., Pettigrove, K., Muftic, D., Beesley, K., Hession, C., & Aisthorpe, B. (2020, April 30). Discharge planning LEAVING checklist for people with aphasia. https://aphasia.org.au AAA

Hersh, D., Worrall, L., Howe, T., Sherratt, S., & Davidson, B. (2012). SMARTER goal setting in aphasia rehabilitation. *Aphasiology*, 26(2): 220–233. https://doi.org/https://doi.org/10.1080/02687038.2011.640392

Hoepner, J. K., Dahl, K. A., Keegan, L. C., & Proud, D. N. (2024). Healthcare perceptions of persons with traumatic brain injuries across providers: shortcomings in the chronic phase of care. *Brain Injury*, 38(5): 347–354. https://doi.org/10.1080/02699052.2024.2311332

James, K. (2011). *The Strands of Speech and Language Therapy: Weaving Plan for Neurorehabilitation*, 1st ed. Routledge. https://doi.org/10.4324/9781003072461

Joseph, S., Becker, S., Elwick, H., & Silburn, R. (2012). Adult carers quality of life questionnaire (AC-QcL): development of an evidence-based tool. *Mental Health Review Journal*, 17(2): 57–69.

Language recovery after stroke: https://aphasialab.org/research

MacDonald, S. (2017). Introducing the model of cognitive-communication competence: a model to guide evidence-based communication interventions after brain injury. *Brain Injury*, 31(13–14): 1760–1780. doi: 10.1080/02699052.2017.1379613

Manning, M., MacFarlane, A., Hickey, A., Galvin, R., & Franklin, S. (2021). 'I hated being ghosted' – The relevance of social participation for living well with post-stroke aphasia: qualitative interviews with working aged adults. *Health Expectations*, 24(4): 1504–1515.

Marsh, E. B., & Hillis, A. E. (2006). Recovery from aphasia following brain injury: the role of reorganization. *Progress in Brain Research*, 157: 143–156.

Morris, J., Franklin, S., & Menger, F. (2011) Returning to work with aphasia: A case study. Aphasiology. 25(8): 890–907. doi: 10.1080/02687038.2010.549568

Murphy, J., & Oliver, T. (2013). The use of talking mats to support people with dementia and their carers to make decisions together. *Health & Social Care in the Community* [online], 21(2): 171–180. https://doi.org/10.1111/hsc.12005

Pearl, G., Sage, K., & Young, A. (2011). Involvement in volunteering: an exploration of the personal experience of people with aphasia. *Disability and Rehabilitation*, 33(19–20): 1305–1821. https://doi.org/10.3109/09638288.2010.549285

Ramanathan, P., Turner, H. A., & Stevens, M. C. (2018). Intensive cognitive rehabilitation therapy for chronic traumatic brain injury:

a case study of neural correlates of functional improvement. *Aphasiology*, 33(3): 289–319. https://doi.org/10.1080/02687038.2018.1461801

Riedeman, S., & Turkstra L. (2018). Knowledge, confidence, and practice patterns of speech language pathologists working with adults with traumatic brain injury. *American Journal of Speech-Language Pathology*, 27(1): 181–191. doi:10.1044/2017_AJSLP-17-0011

Simmons-Mackie, N., Worrall, L., Murray, L. L., Enderby, P., Rose, M. L., Paek, E. J., & Klippi, A. (2016). The top ten: best practice recommendations for aphasia. *Aphasiology*, 31(2): 131–151. https://doi.org/10.1080/02687038.2016.1180662

Turner-Stokes, L. (2009). Goal attainment scaling (GAS) in rehabilitation: a practical guide. *Clinical Rehabilitation*, 23(4): 362–370. https://doi.org/10.1177/0269215508101742

Vestling, M., Tufvesson, B., & Iwarsson, S.(2003). Indicators for return to work after stroke and the importance of work for subjective well-being and life satisfaction. *Journal of Rehabilitation Medicine*, 35(3): 127–131.

Vogel, A., Maruff, P., & Morgan, A. (2010). Evaluation of communication assessment practices during the acute stages post stroke. *Journal of Evaluation in Clinical Practice*, 16(6): 1183–1188.

Volkmer, A. (2013). *Assessment and Therapy for Language and Cognitive Communication Difficulties in Dementia and Other Progressive Diseases*. J&R Press.

Volkmer, A., Alves, E. V., Bar-Zeev, H. et al. (2025). An international core outcome set for primary progressive aphasia (COS-PPA): consensus-based recommendations for communication interventions across research and clinical settings. *Alzheimer's & Dementia*, 21(1): 1–24. https://doi.org/10.1002/alz.14362

Volkmer, A., Walton, H., Swinburn, K., Spector, A., Warren, J. D., & Beeke, S. (2023). Results from a randomised controlled pilot study of the Better Conversations with Primary Progressive Aphasia (BCPPA) communication partner training program for people with PPA and their communication partners. *Pilot and Feasibility Studies*, 9(1): 87. https://doi.org/1186/s40814-023-01301-6

Wade, D. T. (2009). Goal setting in rehabilitation: an overview of what, why and how. *Clinical Rehabilitation*, 23(4): 291–295. https://doi.org/10.1177/0269215509103551

Watila, M. M., & Balarabe, S. A. (2015). Factors predicting post-stroke aphasia recovery. *Journal of the Neurological Sciences,* 352(1–2): 12–18.

Wilson, S. M., Eriksson, D. K., Brandt, T. H., Schneck, S. M., Lucanie, J. M., Burchfield, A. S., Quillen, I. A., de Riesthal, M., Kirshner, H. S., Beeson, P. M., Ritter, L., Kidwell, C. S. (2019). Patterns of recovery from aphasia in the first two weeks after stroke. *Journal of Speech, Language, and Hearing Research,* 62(3): 723–732.

Yamaji, C. and Maeshima, S. (2022). Spontaneous recovery and intervention in aphasia. *Aphasia Compendium.* IntechOpen. doi: 10.5772/intechopen.100851

Chapter 4

ASSESSMENT

33 WHY DO WE ASSESS?

Your assessment is an essential part of your clinical management of someone with aphasia. The purpose of assessment is to:

- make a differential **diagnosis**
- **understand** this person's aphasia
- understand the **impact** of the aphasia on their life
- be able to **explain** aphasia to your client and their family
- establish **baselines**
- inform **management** (including **prognosis** and **goal setting** and **treatment options**).

Diagnosis: You need to know whether someone has aphasia and/or another communication problem and assessment enables you to make a differential diagnosis. You may find other communication problems at assessment, alongside the aphasia, such as speech production or cognitive deficits (see Chapters 5 and 6).

Understanding the nature and severity of the aphasia: What are the linguistic and communicative strengths and weaknesses of your client? How do their language difficulties relate to theoretical frameworks of language processing? Assessment means you can make a hypothesis as to what the underlying language impairments are and, with this, you design appropriate therapy.

The impact: What is the impact of the aphasia on someone's functional communication and on their quality of life? How is the aphasia limiting participation in their daily life and their activities (particularly their work and social life).

Explaining the aphasia: You need an understanding of the nature of this person's aphasia so that you can explain to them and their family what has happened to their communication (see Chapter 3). Assessment can be a good opportunity to provide information and education about aphasia and to explain the purpose of assessment and share the results and implications.

Baselines and outcome measures: Measurements of someone's performance in assessment tasks (e.g. speech in conversation, reading comprehension) provide baselines to evaluate therapy.

Prognosis: Your assessment may inform your prognosis for the possible recovery of someone's aphasia, contributing to goal setting and plans for therapy (see Chapter 3).

Goal setting: Assessment identifies communicative strengths and weaknesses, the impact of the aphasia on the client's participation in everyday life and informs goal setting. Goal setting suggests further assessment and therapy; a client's goals can guide assessment and thus involve the person with aphasia in the assessment process (Hersh et al. 2013). Realistic goals and treatment options can be discussed and agreed in view of the language difficulties revealed by assessment (see Point 21).

Therapy: Often aphasia assessment is focused on identifying the areas with the most profound impairment but a full picture of someone's language strengths and weaknesses is vital in order to have a clear, evidence-based rationale behind the therapy you provide. Remember that a bit more time spent on assessment and using the assessment results to plan therapy means you could target the aphasia more specifically and efficiently; you can plan interventions that are consistent with the nature of the language disorder. Most people with aphasia will have some level of difficulty with comprehension, spontaneous speech, reading and writing, to different degrees; each person presents with a unique profile.

34 PREPARE TO ASSESS

The assessment should include taking a case history, assessing linguistic and cognitive skills and assessing the impact of the aphasia on everyday communication. Gather information before the first appointment so that you spend less time asking questions and more time observing and listening. Start your case history notes and get as much information as you can from the medical notes, referral letter and any relevant reports, and have conversations with other health professionals where appropriate. Look for information about someone's handedness, hearing and vision; undetected problems can make assessment less reliable. Look beyond visual acuity (see Chapter 5). Ask for information from the person with aphasia and their partner/family before the appointment; send a short questionnaire and/or email or phone to check information such as home address, date of birth.

Preparing yourself: Before meeting every new client, it is appropriate to feel a little nervous. You know that every person with aphasia that you meet (and their partner/family) will be different: with their own particular language difficulties and presentation, their own personality and emotional state in response to their changed communication skills. As you become more experienced, try not to lose that slight nervousness. It is telling you to be on your toes and to focus on listening well, ask useful questions (and not too many), with goal setting and therapy in mind. It is an essential part of being a good clinician, no matter how long you have been working with people with aphasia.

35 ASSESSMENT OPTIONS

There is no one set of tests or assessments that are 'the' assessment for people with aphasia. Different assessments take different approaches to the aphasia and have advantages and disadvantages. There are different assessment options that we can use to measure the nature and level of someone's aphasia, its impact on everyday conversation and on life participation. You may have preferences, more knowledge of some assessments and limited resources. Keep updated on assessments as part of your clinical development. Assessment of language is often divided into informal, formal (non-standardised or standardised assessments) and functional communication assessments. (There are also screening tests, assessments of life participation, assessments of psychological well-being, goal attainment scaling, self-rating scales, see Appendix 4.) At an initial appointment the focus is usually on gathering information via an interactive interview and conversation; key parts of an 'informal' assessment. Goals emerge from the initial conversation and point to further assessment. You may do some brief assessment there and then, in light of these goals, or at another appointment.

36 INFORMAL ASSESSMENT

It is not easy to define 'informal assessment'; therapists may have different understandings of why they do it and what it consists of (Thomson et al. 2018). What is generally agreed is that an informal assessment is a 'fluid exercise in critical thinking' and a 'process of creating and manipulating stimuli for the purpose of making clinical decisions, usually by answering hypothesis questions' (Murray & Coppens 2022, pp. 94, 80). It does not have to involve a published assessment, although it might include some more formal tasks, and what goes on in the session may not have the planned, defined steps that either a formal assessment or therapy session might have. There is also a less 'formal' way of interacting with someone in such assessment sessions; which suits an initial appointment; part of the objective of the assessment is to establish a relationship with the client and their family. We also choose tasks such as conversation and narrative descriptions, which are more informal (Hersh, Wood & Armstrong 2018). Informal assessment is very helpful if what we are looking for is a better understanding of someone's ability to communicate in a 'natural' environment (or as near as we can get to one in the context of a therapy session). It also provides an initial sample of someone's language; particularly how they manage in conversation and what their discourse is like. By engaging someone in conversation you are trying to get closer to 'everyday talk'. Informal assessment methods often include:

- observation
- semi-structured, interactive interview
- conversation.

> Before the first appointment, Brenda rang to let me know that her dad was very nervous of being asked a lot of questions that he would find difficult to answer and having to do things he found difficult to do. So, his assessment session was informal and designed in the form of a gentle conversation and getting to know each other. It was possible to learn a great deal about Mr. P's aphasia from this. Brenda contacted me after the appointment to say that her father had really enjoyed the session, and her mother had found it very relaxing.

37 OBSERVATION

It is important to take note of someone's physical state, including their mobility. Are they using a wheelchair, walking unaided or with a stick? Are there signs of paralysis or paresis on one side of the body, legs and/or arms or hands? Are your chairs appropriate and comfortable, with options for arm rests? Notice non-verbal communication; eye-contact, facial expressions. What do these suggest about their level of awareness, fatigue, mood? (See Chapter 5.) During the session, you will be making observations about the person with aphasia and their partner/family. Remember that your observations can be influenced by your expectations of what is likely to occur; so, make sure that you record the conversation, e.g. specific word errors in an answer to a specific question. Try and allow for the impact your observing someone's communication can have on them by observing their conversation with someone else in the session; so promote dialogue between the person with aphasia and their partner.

38 SEMI-STRUCTURED, INTERACTIVE INTERVIEW

It is useful to carry out a semi-structured interview; and you can add to your written case history form along with engaging the client and their family in a conversation and collect a sample of someone's language. The information you get about someone's work history and current job and/or hobbies and interests is useful and relevant to goal planning and therapy. Assessment may include looking at someone's plans and ability to return to work (see Point 23). If the person with aphasia has retired, do they have hobbies and activities that they may want to continue with that require certain levels of speech, understanding, reading and writing? Ask about their living situation and family. Do they live alone, with family or in a residential or nursing home? Knowing who the person with aphasia communicates with on a daily basis is important when looking at what communication situations they face, what their goals may be, how they spend their time. Are they independent or do they need help for everyday activities, or activities of daily living (ADL)? All this information informs the SLT about the communication needs of the person with aphasia and can be used to draw up treatment plans and their content, such as vocabulary and narrative practice.

Be aware and beware of too much of the session becoming you asking questions; aphasia assessment needs to involve the SLT working together with both the person with aphasia and their family/friends; working together includes balancing the time spent speaking by the therapist and the client. So, think about how you interact and create an assessment that fits the person with aphasia in front of you (Ferguson & Armstrong 2004).

39 CONVERSATION

The obvious way to start is as with anyone else you meet for the first time – to have a conversation. This is the most important and most natural form of communication and arguably the most important area we can improve, in terms of helping the person with aphasia to regain their relationships, work, social status, independent functioning in the world. Most people with aphasia and their families want to improve speech for everyday conversation. As the Aphasia Institute says, 'Life's a conversation'. In an assessment, and even in a clinic with a relative stranger (which the SLT is, at this first appointment), it reflects real-life communication better than most language tests. Even when the person with aphasia reports that they were 'never one for chatting', to be deprived of the choice and ability to have a conversation is something most people with aphasia find challenging. Aura Kagan argued that aphasia can mask (obscure) someone's ability to communicate and that this is 'normally revealed through conversation' (Kagan 1995, p. 15). Use conversation to put people at their ease; you might begin the conversation with a greeting, introducing yourself and brief remarks about the weather, or about their journey to clinic. Then a statement to acknowledge why they are here and a question, for example: 'Hello. I am _____. It is good to see you (both/all).' 'Do take a seat/and put your stick by the desk.' 'Isn't it a lovely day/I hope you didn't have too much trouble parking/getting through the rain to get here.' 'I understand you have had (a stroke/a head injury/have a brain tumour) and you are having difficulties with your speech/with communicating. Can you tell me about that?' or 'How can I help?'

Many people with aphasia do not remember much if anything about the stroke or brain injury and can find hearing the account from their partner a difficult or distressing experience. This too can be a time for education about stroke and normalising their lack of memory/awareness of the events. Other people with aphasia appreciate the opportunity to tell the story of what happened, as best they can, to an interested audience. Remember that in a self-report what is said is not usually the whole picture; it will take longer than one appointment to understand the complexities. It is also common for people to misrepresent a problem; perhaps due to cognitive problems, perhaps because they are not yet aware of the implications of the aphasia.

An essential part of an assessment is to find out how the person with aphasia and their partner describe the communication difficulties they experience, what they know about them and how they view the client's aphasia. People have very different levels of understanding of what aphasia is. Notice the words they use or try to use to describe their speech, their conversation. How the partner describes and comments on the person with aphasia and their communication can give you an initial impression of how this family are managing the aphasia. You may get different information from the person with aphasia and their partner. They may have different views or perceptions of the communication difficulties and of the impact of these on the person with aphasia and everyday conversation and activities (Hesketh et al. 2011). This initial informal assessment may suggest significant communication difficulties, and possibly a lack of awareness on the part of the person with the aphasia who may be unaware of how unsuccessful their communication is, so appear untroubled by their aphasia, or insistent that it is just other people being obtuse or unhelpful or deaf.

Some people with aphasia may overestimate and others underestimate the communication difficulties and the impact on everyone's quality of life. The person with aphasia may be frustrated and in a low mood, the partner exasperated and exhausted. All their behaviours in the conversation and responses to questions provide an informal assessment of how the person with aphasia and their partner are managing the changes in communication that the aphasia is causing. Listen to the remarks made by both people carefully and without judgement. If appropriate in this first session, you could ask for more information, so you can begin to appreciate what both the person with aphasia and their partner are dealing with. Normalise the difficult thoughts and feelings that people have in dealing with aphasia if these are expressed (see Points 95–100).

The initial conversation is the beginning of assessing (understanding) the client's communication; and will give you information about their understanding, their spontaneous speech and their response to the changes in communication abilities.

- Note whether they attend to the conversation, to any questions asked, and attempt to speak.
- What do you see in their facial expressions that gives you information?
- Is there any speech and, if so, how much? How fluent is it? Are they getting a message across? Is that message appropriate in the context of this conversation or question asked? Note any word finding difficulties and errors made in speech or writing.
- Are they unaware of their difficulties? Do they try and correct themselves?
- Do they turn to the person with them to answer for them? Does the partner answer before the client has a chance to try?
- What is the response of that partner and how does the person with aphasia respond to their answer? Do they attempt to show agreement or disagreement? Is there turn-taking?

- Do they show an emotional response to not being able to communicate independently, perhaps a tearful or indifferent or frustrated or angry response? (See Point 96.)
- With a pen and paper in front of them and/or offered to them, do they write spontaneously as an alternative to speech? Or draw? Do they attempt gestures?

SUPPORT CONVERSATION

An assessment should provide the person with aphasia with opportunities to show their abilities, as well as their difficulties. Informal assessment can be an introduction to the use of communication strategies (see Chapter 9, Points 82 and 83); encourage use of writing or gesture alongside speech attempts during the informal assessment and normalise this as a legitimate way to communicate in the sessions. Provide a model to the family of how to encourage all forms of communication to get a message across; accept any attempt at speech, ask, 'Can you write that?', 'Can you show me what you mean/what it is?'. Model putting the different forms of communication together to try and understand the message.

Many people with aphasia do not automatically turn to other ways of getting their message across. Note whether they are flexible enough to do so in response to your prompts and models and see what support is helpful. Does writing key words during a conversation support the person with aphasia to understand? Doing so shows both the person with aphasia and their partner that support to communicate is the new normal. The person with aphasia should feel an active participant in assessment, supported to show their strengths as well as supported when their difficulties are apparent. It is important to create or maintain their motivation for therapy. Remember that every aspect of the session can be useful for your information-gathering. An unplanned, unexpected event may give you useful information about the communication preferences and abilities of someone with aphasia.

> Mr. S had significant communication difficulties as a result of his aphasia with almost no spontaneous speech. Early in therapy he showed his ability to spontaneously use gesture, pointing and facial expressions to good effect. Mrs. S started to behave oddly in the session, and he used these means of getting an important message across to the SLT about his wife's increasingly strange behaviour, which was that she had diabetes, and urgently needed the glucose tablets in her bag.

EXPANDING ON CONVERSATION: NARRATIVE AND DISCOURSE

An assessment is a particular and unusual context for anyone to be in, and the language you hear from someone with aphasia is limited by this context. In your attempts to elicit more everyday language it can be helpful to introduce a topic which gives your client an opportunity to produce longer chunks of speech, which means you can see what strengths and weaknesses there are in their language production in conversational speech or discourse. You will begin to discover more about their word retrieval and sentence level difficulties. Start with a topic relevant to them; an immediate one such as the journey to the clinic, perhaps their family, what they do for a living, where they live. Begin, 'Can you tell me about ...?' Look for different kinds of discourse, a monologue, a dialogue. As part of a more formal assessment, you can elicit narrative descriptions by asking someone to tell you about a holiday, their first school and their hobbies; or structured narratives via composite picture descriptions.

WHAT TO DO WITH THE INFORMATION FROM THE CONVERSATION AND DISCOURSE

Does conversation just tell us about someone's functional communication abilities, or can it tell us more about the language impairment (and so be part of a formal assessment)? It is useful to observe and, if possible, record someone with aphasia in conversation with others, to record the discourse during assessment. It is always a challenge for the SLT to put the time aside to evaluate the conversation recorded, to evaluate it and perhaps transcribe it (Armstrong et al. 2007) but it can be beneficial. With experience, and looking at examples in aphasia literature, you will pick out some of the key strengths and weaknesses of someone's conversation and note them for therapy planning (Ramsberger & Rende 2002).

RECORDING A SAMPLE OF SPEECH, WRITING

It is important not to spend a lot of time in the assessment writing notes; you need to pay close attention and listen well to the person with aphasia and their partner. If they have your attention, they are more likely to give you more information. So, with their permission, record an audio and/or visual sample of their conversation. Make some notes of the key points (don't rely on memory) so that you can return to those points later. Ideally, aim to record in different settings, on the ward, in a group, with family and friends, with staff. Get samples of their writing, even if you are not assessing this formally you can ask someone to write their name, or orally spell their name for your records.

40 FORMAL OR STANDARDISED ASSESSMENT

Formal assessments are published tests available to aphasia therapists to use which can assess language impairment, functional activities, participation or quality of life (see Appendix 4 for list of assessments and Further Reading). The assessment, particularly when standardised, is synonymous with a test, which we carry out under controlled conditions in an objective way; be careful to avoid influencing or leading a response.

41 ASSESSMENT OF LANGUAGE IMPAIRMENT

Assessments focus on the details of the language difficulties someone presents with in order to find out about their language impairment; they follow the International Classification of Functioning, Disability and Health (ICF) level of body structure and function (impairment) (WHO 2001). There are a large number of different assessments, including those which consider several areas of language, such as the Boston Diagnostic Aphasia Examination (BDAE) (Goodglass, Kaplan & Barresi 2001) and the Comprehensive Aphasia Test (CAT) (Swinburn, Porter & Howard 2023) and those assessing specific language areas, such as *Pyramids and Palm Trees* (Howard & Patterson 1992), which look at underlying semantic knowledge, the Boston Naming Test (Kaplan 2001), which focuses on spoken word retrieval. There are also pen-and-paper (or online) assessments, where tasks are presented to the client (e.g. picture naming, written word-to-picture matching), which look at someone's language comprehension and production. The tasks assess language processing at different levels; letter/sound, word and sentence, phrase/connected speech or paragraph.

The BDAE (Goodglass et al. 2001) is an example of an assessment battery which diagnoses and classifies people with aphasia according to the syndromes described in Chapter 2, Point 10 (e.g. Broca's, Wernicke's). While these assessment batteries are widely used, it is important to note that they do not provide a theoretical framework to interpret the results and do not consider psycholinguistic variables (properties of words, e.g. frequency, imageability) which we need to design therapy (Bruce & Edmondson 2010). Comprehensive language assessments in use in clinical practice that have a cognitive neuropsychological approach to understanding the aphasia include the Psycholinguistic Assessment of Language Processing in Aphasia (PALPA) (Kay, Lesser & Coltheart, 1992) and the CAT (Swinburn et al. 2023). These give therapists detailed information about the language impairments and the results can be related to a model of language processing which suggests a working hypothesis as to where the language difficulties are. That hypothesis then suggests treatment areas.

Formal tests provide a **structured format** for assessment. They separate out specific skills. Find out in advance how long the test is likely to take; you may need to plan to carry out some parts of the assessment at different appointments. Be discerning, read the test manual, which should give you a clear rationale for the test and tell you how the test was developed, how the items in it were chosen, what other tests it is similar to, what it measures, e.g. written sentence comprehension, what qualifications you need to carry out the test and understand the results and whether you need particular training to carry it out. It should also tell you how the scores your client gets relate to norms and the lowest and highest scores of 'controls' (people who are a good 'match' for your clients, e.g. similar age), provide useful information about how to present the test, time limits and how you should respond to someone's answers and how to score the test results. An assessment should set out clearly how to interpret the results. The results should give you useful information about the underlying nature of someone's aphasia, relating to a language processing model.

Assessments of language impairment can also provide useful information about someone's everyday communication, with studies showing that scores on picture naming relate to the ability to retrieve nouns in everyday conversation (Herbert et al. 2008); there are also assessments that aim to measure communication in a functional context.

42 ASSESSMENT OF FUNCTIONAL COMMUNICATION

The ICF framework for defining aphasia (WHO 2001) describes areas which need to be assessed in order to plan effective therapy beyond measuring language (and cognitive) abilities; functional 'real world' communication sits across both the levels of activity and participation. Assessments of functional communication look to assess how the aphasia affects someone's ability to function in everyday life and their quality of life, e.g. the Stroke and Aphasia Quality of Life Scale (Hilari et al. 2003).

Assessments of functional communication look at how someone is using language in everyday communication contexts, rather than focusing on the language impairment. They assume that assessments that isolate language functions cannot tell us everything we need to know to design therapy to improve everyday communication. The ICF framework can guide the assessment methods focusing on the activity limitations and participation restrictions the aphasia brings. Formal assessments of the consequences of the aphasia, i.e. limits on participation and activities, include assessing the impact of living with aphasia (e.g. Swinburn et al. 2023) and self-rating their abilities to perform everyday tasks (Frattali 1995). Ideally, there is assessment in context where we consider the assessment of functional communication abilities within the environment someone lives in (Do they live alone? Are they able to communicate if there were an emergency?).

43 ASSESSMENT AS PART OF THERAPY

There is so much to assess and so many aspects of someone's communication to take into account that rather than thinking of assessment and therapy as being separate and sequential, it is helpful to think of assessment as part of therapy, something that carries on throughout the therapeutic journey. You build on the knowledge you gather from whatever assessment is possible and realistic in one session. You will assess the same or different language areas later, and later assessment may add to or revise a hypothesis about someone's aphasia and with it the therapy focus. Assessment is an ongoing part of therapy; therapy may target a goal set by someone with aphasia and during the therapy it may become clear that there is a need to know more about their skills and deficits in a particular area (e.g. writing or turn-taking in conversation) in order for therapy to be appropriately provided/directed to reach that goal.

> Assessment can often follow issues about communication that your client or their family bring up from their everyday lives. During a structured conversation, the husband of a client with aphasia said that 'W wants to

> read her many emails, but when she tries, she doesn't seem to understand them.' I suggested we look at her reading in more detail ('we can have a look at that in an assessment'), and W was keen to do so.

Assessment can be an introduction to therapy, providing a model for the SLT sessions. While your aim is to find out information and get data to make your initial hypothesis about this person's aphasia, it is important to set up the therapy space so that it creates a working relationship with your client and their partner or family. Make it an extended conversation about communication. Such an atmosphere makes it more likely that any assessment tasks you present will be more readily accepted. That way you will find out more about the impact of the aphasia on their everyday life. This helps to establish that therapy is a collaborative process and that the key players are the person with aphasia, their partner, their family and the therapist. It also emphasises that the work to improve communication continues when they head out of the therapy room. Only they can do the repetitive work of therapy tasks, only they can practise supported conversation together and it will be them dealing with the bus driver or going back to work with changed communication skills. You have an opportunity to show that SLT assessment is done to provide appropriate therapy and support; it is not an interrogation or series of tests, but a joint exploration to understand the aphasia that only begins at this first appointment.

Assessment is an introduction to working with a therapist. Take time to prepare a structured and well-planned first appointment so your client has confidence that you are a professional who understands aphasia, the rehabilitation process and wants to find out what is important to them in terms of communication. Do not think that means you have to present yourself as all-knowing; it is fine to say that you are not sure, or you don't know, and you will find out. And then find out.

There are excellent resources for clinicians to access support with providing aphasia therapy, see Appendix 5 for a list of these organisations and links.

44 IMPACT OF ASSESSMENT

Who learns what from assessment? All forms of assessment are hugely beneficial for the SLT, and we rely on the evidence of informal and formal assessments to learn about someone's aphasia and goals and to begin to plan treatments. At best, assessment can be a learning opportunity for the client. It needs to be something that the client understands; both what is happening and why and then the results and implications of an assessment. Remember that any assessment is only a snapshot of the person at that moment on that day. The assessment environment may not enable them to reveal a full picture of their communication ability. Remember the impact of aphasia can vary from day to day. So, balance what you see at assessment with reports from the person with aphasia and their family and repeat assessments to get a more informative baseline. So, as well as asking questions, be prepared to answer them. Make the link between assessment and goals clear. This helps to make assessment a powerful motivator for learning and engagement in therapy.

Even while you make the assessment session as joint an endeavour as you can, it is also appropriate for you to guide the session to make sure that the time spent is informative and useful for everyone. Lead the session, observing and taking someone from initial conversation through a variety of tasks, when appropriate, with purpose and confidence. Remember to explain assessments clearly, including the need for all responses, including errors; and that assessment will often highlight difficulties. The emotional impact of the spotlight on deficits on someone with aphasia (and their partner) is something that needs monitoring and you may need to adjust what you do or how much you do in an assessment in response to the reactions that assessment can give rise to. Some people can be particularly aware of how you are evaluating their responses; perhaps wanting to look at what you are writing or be crestfallen at the sight of the ticks and crosses on the record sheets. Depending on the client, you can explain the errors, remind them how important they are (see 'She's getting everything wrong') or keep the record sheet out of sight. In any assessment, try and balance the time spent with you asking questions, or asking for responses, with time in more natural conversation.

45 SOME COMMON ISSUES AROUND ASSESSMENT

'It's such mild aphasia, nothing seems wrong' It is possible for an assessment to show few significant problems, in terms of assessment scores. But this is not the only factor in making clinical judgements as to whether therapy is indicated. Assessment needs to consider key factors such as someone's ability to get their message across in good time (so you should note the delays in speech, time how long it takes them to describe the Cookie Theft (Goodglass et al. 2001) picture, for example, delays in writing and how often they have to correct errors). Some assessments have delays and self-corrections acknowledged in the score sheets so you should note these and take them into account. Either during a conversation, or listening to the recording of a conversation, measure the time it takes the person with aphasia to have their say. Someone's scores may be high, but the impact of the word retrieval difficulties, reduced fluency and their response to their changed communication abilities may include a lack of confidence, distress and despair. So, it is even more important to measure the impact of the aphasia on their lives, including on their quality of life and the psychological impact. Assessing the impact of the aphasia includes finding out how significant a problem it is for that person. Someone's assessment may include meaningful, fluent conversation and good scores in tasks, but the person with aphasia may experience their communication difficulties as significantly disabling and/or upsetting, preventing them from working, from having their say in conversation. There is no simple correlation between test scores and severity; the impact of the aphasia on someone's participation in everyday life should be taken into account when deciding on therapy.

'But he understands everything, so why are you assessing his comprehension?' You will often find that the family say that the person with aphasia 'understands everything'. Often the family tends to focus on speech production and not on difficulties with understanding. Sometimes this is connected to a desire to present their loved one as competent (and not someone with dementia or a psychological problem, which is what people often associate with not understanding). People with aphasia also try to cover up not understanding. You may find that when you assess comprehension, the partner will insist that the words are not ones that the person with aphasia would have known before, or your accent is putting them off, or, anyway, what does this have to do with their speech? So, assessment of comprehension needs to be introduced carefully. Normalise comprehension difficulties as part of aphasia; distinct from memory problems and to do with language processing not intellect. Introduce assessment as a set of tasks which may be quite easy or a bit demanding but important because with the results of the tasks tell us all something about the aphasia and about how best to treat it so that the person with aphasia can get back to having conversations. Sometimes assessment of comprehension shows up significant difficulties which someone with aphasia may have some awareness of but is adept at covering up in everyday conversation.

Peter talked a lot in the assessment, and it was a jovial conversation where he apologised a lot for the word retrieval difficulties and word errors he made in speech.

> It became clear that he may have kept talking because that was easier than listening; his lack of appropriate responses to questions certainly suggested that he was finding it difficult to understand what was said to him (and later assessment showed difficulties processing auditory information, including at a single word level). It took some time for both Peter and his wife to realise that the aphasia had caused significant problems with his understanding. The realisation began at the first appointment, in an informal assessment, by the therapist allowing the difficulties following the structured conversation and questions to become obvious without saying anything about them specifically. Once they both acknowledged the comprehension difficulties in conversation, (made easier once they had some understanding of aphasia) he accepted the need for therapy that targeted his auditory processing skills and strategies for managing in conversation. This treatment brought improvements in his understanding of what was said to him and in his self-monitoring of his speech production. Peter began to have more success in getting his message across in conversation; as he monitored his output better, he was able to self-correct, to pause, to use writing to clarify his understanding of words and to ask his conversation partner to help.

'She's getting everything wrong' It is difficult to watch people fail at tasks, but there is a way to manage this and still carry out an assessment.

- Present the assessment as a 'fact finding mission'. Use phrases like; "I'm going to ask you to do some different things; we'll talk about some pictures. I'll ask you tell me about some of them, there'll be some reading and writing.

Some of the things I ask you to do will be straight-forward, some will be easy for you to do, and others will be more difficult. Everything you do will tell us what is going on with your speech, your reading. Any mistakes you make give us useful information about what's happened to your language. If you can't do something, that's useful to know. What happens when you try is important information. Errors tell us more about your aphasia. We need to know what you can do and what is more difficult so we can work out how to improve it".

- Many formal assessments have a 'cut-off'; if someone is unable to make any response on e.g. four consecutive items, you can finish that task. You can apply that idea of a 'cut-off' to other assessments.
- There is usually something that your client will find some success doing in the assessment. Look for it and highlight it. Try and end the assessment on a task that they have more success with. You need to hold onto the broader picture; to focus on what constitutes success for your client in the long term; improved communication, helped by well-founded therapy which depends on thorough formal assessment of their language at the same time as finding a way to prevent them from becoming disheartened.

'He has such severe aphasia it's impossible to assess him' It is possible for someone's aphasia to be so severe that it is very difficult to carry out any kind of assessment.

- It is still possible to get some baseline of their abilities via observation or by trying therapy tasks. You may need to start both assessment and therapy with object matching or picture matching activities. Assessment starting at this level should alert you to possible issues with fatigue, attention, concentration, neglect, object or picture recognition disorders and the need for other assessments (e.g. Riddoch 1993). See Chapter 5.

- Use supported conversation techniques (see Chapter 14) and the pictures from the Aphasia Institute, for example, to try and elicit conversations.

'I don't have time to do much assessment' There may be service restrictions and time pressures that make it a challenge to do the appropriate assessments. You may work in a health service organisation that asks you to cover a large caseload on wards or outpatient clinics and/or offers a fixed number of therapy sessions. You may have to divide your time between managing communication and swallowing disorders. You may be treating clients whose health insurance company limits the number of therapy sessions they can have, or people who have a limited budget for therapy. In these situations, there may be pressure on you to limit the amount of time you spend on assessment. In some parts of the UK, the limited amount of time offered to people with aphasia for therapy can mean that of what is often 6 sessions routinely provided, 2 may be taken up with assessment. While two sessions may be adequate for some assessments (e.g. the CAT; Swinburn 2023) there may be other assessments that are needed in order to adequately understand the nature of someone's aphasia. With limited time, assessments must be useful for the person with aphasia and their partner and family. So, choose assessments carefully and make the assessment sessions therapeutic. You may be challenged about how much time you spend on assessment. You could make the case that time spent on assessment means that you can target therapy more appropriately and efficiently to meet the needs of the person with aphasia; and will be able to establish baselines and evaluate the benefits of therapy too. There is "no substitute for a detailed, rigorous assessment of the patient's condition that allows more target-specific therapy" (Lum 2002)

46 AFTER THE ASSESSMENT

Remember that assessment, whatever form it takes, can only be a partial reflection of someone's ability to communicate. We do our best to assess in different ways and to take the results of the qualitative interview, the informal observations and formal assessments and begin to build a picture of someone's strengths and weaknesses, their goals and psychological reactions to the aphasia. From that picture we make a hypothesis about what areas of language it would be helpful to target in therapy to work towards the goals identified. Repeat the same assessments you used to diagnose the aphasia at the end of their therapy to measure change in someone's communication abilities; in this way you can measure any success of therapy for that person.

REPORTING ON THE ASSESSMENT

Give your client the results of their assessments. A summary in the session is part of the discussion about next steps. Remember that 40–80 per cent of health care information is forgotten immediately (Kessels 2003) so provide an accessible written report. Use an aphasia-friendly format (using key written words and perhaps pictures or icons) so it can be used by the person with aphasia and their family at home. With the permission of the person with aphasia, send the report to the referring clinician (often a consultant), GP and relevant health care professionals (e.g. occupational therapist, nurse specialist) to inform them of the assessment findings, and what therapy is being offered. The report is an important part of your professional profile so spend time making sure it is accurate, to the point and without grammatical or spelling errors.

REFERENCES

Armstrong, L., Brady, M., Mackenzie, C., & Norrie, J. (2007) Transcription-less analysis of aphasic discourse: a clinician's dream or a possibility? *Aphasiology*, 21(3–4): 355–374. doi: 10.1080/02687030600911310

Bruce, C. and Edmonson, A. (2010). Letting the CAT out of the bag: a review of the Comprehensive Aphasia Test. Commentary on

Howard, Swinburn, and Porter, 'Putting the CAT out: what the Comprehensive Aphasia Test has to offer us'. *Aphasiology*, 24(1): 79–93.

Ferguson, A., & Armstrong, E. (2004). Reflections on speech-language therapists' talk: implications for clinical practice and education. *International Journal of Language and Communication Disorders*, 39(4): 469–507. doi:10.1080/1368282042000226879

Frattali, C. M., Thompson, C. K., Holland, A. L. et al. (1995). *American Speech-Language-Hearing Association Functional Assessment of Communication Skills for Adults (ASHAFACS)*. American Speech-Language-Hearing Association (ASHA).

Herbert, R., Hickin, J., & Howard, D., Osborne, F., & Best, W. (2008). Do picture-naming tests provide a valid assessment of lexical retrieval in conversation in aphasia? *Aphasiology*, 22(2): 184–203. doi: 10.1080/02687030701262613

Hersh, D., Worrall, L., O'Halloran, R., Brown, K., Grohn, B., & Rodriguez, A. (2013). Assess for success: evidence for therapeutic assessment. In N. Simmons-Mackie, J. M. King, & D. R. Beukelman (Eds.), *Supporting Communication for Adults with Acute and Chronic Aphasia* (pp.145–164). Paul H. Brookes Publishing Co., Inc. www.brookespublishing.com

Hersh, D., Wood, P., & Armstrong, E. (2018) Informal aphasia assessment, interaction and the development of the therapeutic relationship in the early period after stroke, *Aphasiology*, 32(8): 876–901. https://doi.org/10.1080/02687038.2017.1381878

Hesketh, A., Long, A., & Bowen, A. on behalf of the ACTNoW Research Study. (2011). Agreement on outcome: speaker, carer, and therapist perspectives on functional communication after stroke. *Aphasiology*, 25(3): 291–308.

Hilari, K., Byng, S., Lamping, D. L., & Smith, S. C. (2003). Stroke and Aphasia Quality of Life Scale-39 (SAQOL-39): evaluation of acceptability, reliability, and validity. *Stroke*, 34(8): 1944–1950. https://doi.org/10.1161/01.STR.0000087987.46660.ED

Kagan, A. (1995). Revealing the competence of aphasic adults through conversation: a challenge to health professionals. *Topics in Stroke Rehabilitation*, 2(1): 15–28.

Kay, J., Lesser, R., & Coltheart, M. (1992) *Psycholinguistic Assessments of Language Processing in Aphasia (PALPA)*. Lawrence Erlbaum Associates.

Kessels, R. P. (2003). Patients' memory for medical information. *Journal of the Royal Society of Medicine*, 96(5): 219–222. doi: 10.1177/014107680309600504.

Morris, J., & Webster, J. (2018) Language assessment in aphasia: an international survey of practice, *Aphasiology*, 32(sup1): 149–151. doi: 10.1080/02687038.2018.1485846

Murray, L., & Coppens, P. (2022). Formal and informal assessment of aphasia. In I. Papathanasiou, P. Coppens, & C. Potagas (Eds.), *Aphasia and Related Neurogenic Communication Disorders*, 3rd ed. (pp. 79–108). Jones and Bartlett Learning.

Ramsberger, G., & Rende, B. (2002). Measuring transactional success in the conversation of people with aphasia. *Aphasiology*, 16(3): 337–353.

Riddoch, M. J., & Humphreys, G. W. (1993). *The Birmingham Object Recognition Battery* (BORB). Erlbaum.

Thomson, J., Gee, M., Sage, K., & Walker, T. (2018). What 'form' does informal assessment take? A scoping review of the informal assessment literature for aphasia. *International Journal of Language & Communication Disorders*, 53(4): 659–674. https://doi.org/10.1111/1460-6984.12382

World Health Organisation (WHO). (2001). *International Classification of Functioning, Disability and Health (WHO-ICF)*. WHO.

FURTHER READING

Bruce, C., & Edmonson, A. (2010). Letting the CAT out of the bag: a review of the Comprehensive Aphasia Test. Commentary on Howard, Swinburn, and Porter, 'Putting the CAT out: what the Comprehensive Aphasia Test has to offer us'. *Aphasiology*, 24(1): 79–93.

Goodglass, H., Kaplan, E., & Barresi, B. (2001). *Boston Diagnostic Aphasia Examination (BDAE)*, 3rd ed. Pearpartner.

Hersh, D., & Boud, D. (2024). Reassessing assessment: what can post stroke aphasia assessment learn from research on assessment in education? *Aphasiology*, 38(1): 123–143. doi: 10.1080/02687038.2022.2163462

Howard, D. & Patterson, K. (1992). *Pyramids and Palm Trees : A Test of Semantic Access from Words to Pictures*. Thames Valley Test Company.

Kaplan, E., Goodglass, H., & Weintraub, S. (2000). *Boston Naming Test*. Williams & Wilkins.

Lum, C. (2002). *Scientific Thinking in Speech and Language Therapy*. Lawrence Erlbaum Associates.

Swinburn, K., Porter, G., & Howard, D. (2023). *The Comprehensive Aphasia Test (CAT)*, 2nd ed. Routledge.

Chapter 5

APHASIA AND COGNITIVE IMPAIRMENTS

47 LANGUAGE AND COGNITION

Language does not operate in isolation from other cognitive processes. Brain lesions often result in damage to executive functions, attention and memory alongside the aphasia and add to the language processing difficulties, to someone's capacity to benefit from therapy; and are important predictors of the quality of life (QOL) of people with aphasia (Nicholas, Hunsaker & Guarino 2017). The question of how language and cognitive abilities are related is complex, particularly thinking and reasoning, and there is no neat correlation between someone's (non-verbal) cognitive ability and language ability. We cannot assume that someone with poor comprehension and/or speech output necessarily has difficulty with other cognitive skills; or that someone with a high level of both comprehension and speech does not have any cognitive difficulties (Marinelli et al. 2017). There are people with aphasia who have impaired language but intact cognitive skills for other everyday functioning.

Language is used both for communication with others and for our own thought processes, which we experience when we think through options or possibilities using inner speech. Whether inner speech is the thought, or language enables the thought is still debated. Clinically, it is helpful to remember that essentially, someone else's thoughts and inner language is very difficult to gauge, perhaps unknowable. However disordered their language may appear to be in conversation and from an assessment, do not make assumptions about underlying cognitive competence and functioning, including inner language and thinking but look at what assessments tell you (see Point 52).

48 EXECUTIVE FUNCTIONS

Executive functions include selective attention, working memory, self-monitoring, initiation, inhibition and cognitive flexibility; importantly, these functions also coordinate different cognitive and communication processes. Impaired executive functions can reduce someone's ability to learn and then apply communication strategies appropriately. Therapy needs to take into account and adapt to any cognitive deficits (see Chapter 10). The ability to repair speech or writing attempts in conversations, for example, requires cognitive flexibility (being able to move between actions and ideas, remember and apply strategies). Other executive functions include reasoning (e.g. making comparisons) and problem solving (e.g. analysing information); all important in language processing.

49 ATTENTION

The ability to focus on incoming information, select one stimulus, ignore others and sustain that focus can be impaired following damage to the left hemisphere of the brain. As well as someone's underlying attention abilities, different communication situations will demand more from attention skills. Attention deficits can affect different aspects of language processing, e.g. auditory comprehension (particularly understanding long chunks of information). Many people with aphasia report finding one-to-one conversations easier than being part of a group. This can reflect difficulties with auditory attention as well as auditory comprehension deficits. **Neglect:** Unilateral neglect is a spatial disorder involving inattention to visual/auditory/tactile stimuli on one side of the body, usually the opposite side to the brain lesion. It is more common following right hemisphere and middle cerebral artery lesions. People may ignore people and objects on the affected side, miss parts of words when reading and parts of drawings when copying. **Hemianopia** is a loss of part of the visual field, following brain lesions that damage visual processing systems. It affects around 30 per cent of people after a stroke. There may be spontaneous recovery, and around 15 per cent of people will recover their full visual field in the first weeks after a stroke, but it can persist for months. Visual neglect and hemianopia can occur together or separately; both can have a significant impact on someone's independent living, e.g. on reading and/or driving.

50 MEMORY

Cognitive functions rely on an ability to retain information. Short-term memory (STM) briefly stores partially processed information. Working memory (WM) temporarily stores information and manipulates it; playing an important role in communication, e.g. tracking what has been said in conversation, what we are about to say, what we read or what we are planning to write. After a traumatic brain injury (TBI), memory impairments are seen in 20–79 per cent of people (depending on factors such as the severity of the TBI) and WM deficits contribute to problems with auditory comprehension of inference or ambiguous information, with understanding discourse and reading comprehension.

51 SPEED OF PROCESSING

As well as processing the language in a conversation (perhaps the interactions of several people), we need to process information when reading from facial expressions and gestures at an appropriate rate. One cognitive-communication deficit after a TBI may be slower processing of tasks, particularly ones that may be demanded in a typical work situation.

52 ASSESSMENT

Because cognitive skills underpin the complex language tasks we work on, we need to have an understanding of someone's cognitive abilities when assessing, planning and delivering aphasia therapy. For many SLTs, there is limited time and difficulty in accessing appropriate assessments. Remember that assessment can be informal, initially based on clinical observations, e.g. is this person alert, making eye contact or responding to conversation, showing signs of fatigue, trying to reduce stimuli by closing their eyes? What are the cognitive demands of the therapy task? Are there simple tasks that highlight which cognitive processes are working well, and which are impaired? Formal assessments may be carried out by a neuropsychologist in a multi-disciplinary team (MDT), with standardised, neuropsychological assessments that can inform communication therapy. Where possible, work collaboratively with the neuropsychologist, sharing results and discussing assessment findings and their implications for therapy (Constantinidou et al. 2012).

ASSESSMENT OF ATTENTION

It is essential to observe whether someone can focus on/attend to incoming spoken/written information the first time you meet someone. There are formal assessments, e.g. the Test of Everyday Attention which looks at selective, alternating and sustained attention (see Appendix 4).

ASSESSMENT OF NEGLECT

Neglect is normally assessed by clinical observation, reports from the person affected and/or their family, pen-and-paper tests and behavioural assessment tools, note assessments by neurologists or ophthalmologists.

ASSESSMENT OF MEMORY

One standardised assessment of STM in people with aphasia which is comprehensive and easy to administer is the Temple Assessment of Language and Short-Term Memory in Aphasia (TALSA) which includes language tasks with different levels of increasing demand on STM (Martin 2018). Remember that many people with aphasia and/or their family refer to their word retrieval difficulties as not being able to 'remember' a word, and it may be important to differentiate between the two.

> Mrs. P described her word retrieval difficulties as not being able to 'remember' a word. She said that this was how she experienced the times when the word was not available; she said, 'there's nothing there' or gestured a wall coming down in front of her. Mr. and Mrs. P were worried that she had 'lost' the words. People assume that if the problem is about memory, there is little hope for change and so not much point in working to improve things. Importantly for how someone with aphasia is treated by others, a problem with memory is conflated into 'losing your marbles' and being a less competent adult. It is therefore important to address the question of memory vs. word retrieval difficulties in your therapy, including education about aphasia, the difference between word retrieval and memory, the nature of word retrieval difficulties (inherently variable and frustrating), discussion about what someone's own difficulties look like, the potential for improvement. Mrs. P found this approach useful and it helped her to engage in regular, targeted therapy for her word retrieval difficulties in clinic and at home and to explain the problems to family and friends.

TESTING SPEED OF PROCESSING

Assessment of communication should measure not only how accurately but also how quickly and efficiently someone is able to process and respond in tasks/conversation. Improving the speed of responses can be an important goal of therapy.

53 TREATMENTS

APHASIA THERAPY

There is evidence that treating the aphasia can improve some cognitive functions including attention, reasoning and executive functions (Marinelli et al. 2017). As part of your aphasia therapy, **education** should include helping someone with aphasia and their family to understand cognitive difficulties and their impact on conversation, on other activities and **advice** on how to focus someone's attention before speaking to them, for example, to promote more successful conversations.

TREATING COGNITIVE DEFICITS

Treatment of impaired attention and executive functions in people with aphasia (including in people many years post-onset) can result in measurable changes in those skills and in the success of conversation (Ramsberger 2005). There is good evidence for treatment of cognitive deficits after **acquired brain injury (ABI)** including errorless learning, training in metacognitive strategies and group therapy. There is evidence to support interventions for verbal reasoning and problem solving to improve communication competence (Kennedy et al. 2008).

MEMORY TREATMENTS

Different approaches to the treatment of memory deficits by SLTs include external memory aids, internal memory strategies, systematic instruction and errorless learning and prospective memory training. The treatment of STM/WM deficits (which may include word/non-word repetition, sentence repetition, picture description) can lead to improvements in spoken sentence and discourse comprehension, everyday communication and reading in some studies. Some treatments focus on cognitive skills (see Further Reading below).

THERAPY FOR ATTENTION DEFICITS

Therapy to improve attention can result in improvements in everyday communication. Therapies include training attention skills and learning metacognitive strategies. Metacognition is the awareness of our own thinking, of what skills we are using, what we are trying to do. Developing this skill in people with aphasia helps them to regulate different cognitive processes.

NEGLECT

There is a lack of evidence for treatments to help people adapt to/manage visual neglect after stroke. Visual scanning training could help manage hemianopia (a visual field deficit with a loss of vision for stimuli in the visual field opposite the site of the brain lesion).[1] Tactus® Apps have a visual attention Therapy app which tests for (left sided) neglect and provides practice scanning for target symbols or letters. In assessments and therapy, it can be helpful to place a bright red card next to the page or picture being used in order to encourage attention to the affected side. If this is helpful, it is a strategy that someone can use when reading.

DRAWING ATTENTION TO THE APHASIA/ACKNOWLEDGING

Often in our assessment and therapy we are drawing attention to what someone cannot do. While this is a necessary part of assessment and therapy, we need to ensure that our client understands why it is necessary, be aware of its impact on their self-esteem and notice their reactions. People often avoid focusing on difficulties. You may wonder if someone really doesn't want to read anything anymore or whether they do not want to acknowledge the new reading difficulties they have. It is important for engagement in therapy to be able to attend to/acknowledge both strengths and weaknesses and you can model this in the way you attend to and/or comment on both. Do you acknowledge successes in conversation? Can you model accepting how communication is in that moment without judgement, including the difficulties, errors, swearing that might occur, so that therapy becomes somewhere that difficulties can be focused on and addressed with non-judgemental curiosity and acceptance? Can you wait, and decide when is a good moment to suggest and/or show other ways to get a message across? Paying attention to something can then be a collaborative and less starkly difficult process.

54 COGNITIVE-COMMUNICATION DISORDERS

Cognitive-communication disorders involve difficulties in communication 'that result from underlying cognitive impairments (attention, memory, organization, information processing, problem solving, and executive functions)' (McDonald et al. 2017). Often these are people with communication difficulties after an ABI or with right hemisphere brain damage (see Chapter 6, Point 58) and/or people with dementia. Alongside communication difficulties, these cognitive impairments add to the difficulties with activities of daily living, social interaction, ability to learn and to work.

55 COVID-19

There is an increased risk of stroke with acute COVID-19 infection, and therefore of aphasia. Cognitive and communication impairments can also be a significant, long-term consequence of having the COVID-19 infection (estimates range from 43–66% for those hospitalised, while 25 per cent of people who were not admitted to hospital reported speech and language problems) (Cummings 2023). So, you are likely to see people with what in 2021 the World Health Organisation defined as a 'post COVID-19 condition' or Long Covid. Beyond obvious causes of brain lesions (stroke, hypoxia), it is not clear what leads to symptoms such as reduced verbal fluency, difficulties with word finding and word errors in speech and reading and writing difficulties. People report experiencing 'brain fog' to describe their cognitive issues such as slower processing speed, poor attention, memory problems, difficulties problem solving. This 'brain fog' may only become apparent when physical symptoms begin to improve, particularly when someone goes back to everyday life and roles, such as work, with the increased cognitive and communication demands.

ASSESSMENT

There are currently no standardised assessments for people with communication changes after COVID-19. You can use assessments such as the Comprehensive Aphasia Test (CAT) (Swinburn, Porter & Howard 2023) and those used with people following ABI. The profile of the deficits may be more similar to what we see in someone's communication following ABI than aphasia after stroke. It is useful to assess discourse (see Appendix 4). On assessment you may also see dysarthria (a motor speech disorder, involving slower and weaker movements of the muscles needed to produce both speech and voice, see Point 57), stammering and even foreign accent syndrome.

REFERRAL

Refer the client on to the appropriate services (e.g. neuropsychology, memory clinic, occupational therapy) for further cognitive assessment and treatment. Support may be available from Long or Post COVID services and/or local support groups. Try and get support yourself from other SLTs working with this client group to develop skills.

THERAPY

Therapy that is helpful includes education about the communication and cognitive difficulties and the causes (differentiating between COVID-19 and dementia, which is often feared; be careful to take a good case history and ask about other medical issues, and make sure you do a thorough assessment in order not to miss possible other causes). Increased understanding helps to manage the frustration and embarrassment. Impairment based therapy may be useful, e.g. for word retrieval, with the objective of improving speed of access to a set of words the client uses frequently. Compensatory therapy may include use of other modalities to get their message across, such as use of memory aids, prompts, diaries. Environmental therapy includes communication partner training for family and friends to improve conversation and support to return to work.

DELIVERY

Delivery of therapy may be by both face-to-face and telehealth. Bear in mind the need to reduce fatigue from travelling to clinic and the fatigue from using screens.

NOTE

1 Randomised controlled trial of Scanning Eye training as a Rehabilitation Choice for Hemianopia after stroke (SEARCH) University of Liverpool, Principal investigator: Professor Fiona Rowe (2023).

REFERENCES

Constantinidou F, Wertheimer, J. C., Tsanadis, J., Evans, C. & Paul, D. R. (2012). Assessment of executive functioning in brain injury: collaboration between speech-language pathology and neuropsychology for an integrative neuropsychological perspective. *Brain Injury*, 26(13–14): 1549–1563. doi: 10.3109/02699052.2012.698786

Cummings, L. (2023) Cognitive-linguistic difficulties in adults with Long COVID. In L. Cummings (Ed.), *COVID-19 and Speech-Language Pathology* (pp. 72–95). Routledge.

Fedorenko, E., & Varley, R. (2016). Language and thought are not the same thing: evidence from neuroimaging and neurological patients. *Annals of New York Academy of Sciences*, 1369(1): 132–153. doi: 10.1111/nyas.13046

Frankel, T., Penn, C., & Ormond-Brown, D. (2007). Executive dysfunction as an explanatory basis for conversation symptoms of aphasia: a pilot study. *Aphasiology*, 21(6–8): 814–828. https://doi.org/10.1080/02687030701192448

Helm-Estabrooks, N. (2002). Cognition and aphasia: a discussion and a study. *Journal of Communication Disorders*, 35(2): 171–186. doi: 10.1016/S0021-9924(02)00063-1.

Kennedy, M. R. T., Coelho, C., Turkstra, L., Ylvisaker, M., Moore, S. M., Yorkston, K., Chiou, H.-H., & Kan, P.-F. (2008). Intervention for executive functions after traumatic brain injury: a systematic review, meta-analysis and clinical recommendations. *Neuropsychological Rehabilitation*, 18(3): 257–299. doi:10.1080/09602010701748644

Marinelli, C. V., Spaccavento, S., Craca, A., Marangolo, P., Angelelli, P. (2017). Different cognitive profiles of patients with severe aphasia. *Behavioural Neurology*, 3(1–15): 3875954. doi: 10.1155/2017/3875954

Martin, N., Minkina, I., Kohen, F. P., & Kalinyak-Fliszar, M. (2018). Assessment of linguistic and verbal short-term memory components of language abilities in aphasia. *Journal of* Neurolinguistics, 48(3–4): 199–225. doi:10.1016/j.jneuroling.2018.02.006

McDonald, S., Gowland, A., Randall, R., Fisher, A., Osborne-Crowley, K., & Honan, C. (2014). Cognitive factors underpinning poor expressive communication skills after traumatic brain injury: theory of mind or executive function? *Neuropsychology*, 28(5): 801–811.

Miyake, A., Emerson, M. J., Friedman N. P. (2000). Assessment of executive functions in clinical settings: problems and recommendations. *Seminars in Speech and Language*, 21(2): 169–183.

Nicholas, M., Hunsaker, E., & Guarino, A. J. (2017). The relation between language, non-verbal cognition and quality of life in people with aphasia. *Aphasiology*, 31(6): 688–702. doi: 10.1080/02687038.2015.1076927

Olsson, C., Arvidsson, P., & Johansson, B. M. (2019). Relations between executive function, language, and functional communication in severe aphasia, *Aphasiology*, 33(7): 821–845. doi: 10.1080/02687038.2019.1602813

O'Neil-Pirozzi, T. M., Kennedy, M., Sohlberg, M. M. (2015). Evidence based practice for the use of internal strategies as a memory compensation technique after brain injury: a systematic review. *The Journal of Head Trauma Rehabilitation*, 31(4): E1–E11. doi:10.1097/HTR.0000000000000181

Peach, R. K., Nathan, M. R., & Beck, K. M. (2017). Language-specific attention treatment for aphasia: description and preliminary findings. *Seminars in Speech and Language*, 38(1): 5–16. https://doi.org/10.1055/s-0036-1597260

Ponsford, J., Bayley, M., Wiseman-Hakes, C., Togher, L., Velikonja, D., McIntyre, A., Janzen, S., & Tate, R. (2014). INCOG recommendations for management of cognition following traumatic brain Injury, Part II: attention and speed of information processing. *The Journal of Head Trauma Rehabilitation*, 29(4): 321–337. doi:10.1097/HTR.0000000000000072

Ramsberger, G. (2005). Achieving conversational success in aphasia by focusing on non-linguistic cognitive skills: a potentially promising new approach, *Aphasiology*, 19(10–11): 1066–1073. doi: 10.1080/02687030544000254

Salis, C., Kelly, H., & Code, C. (2015). Assessment and treatment of short-term and working memory impairments in stroke aphasia: a practical tutorial. *International Journal of Language & Communication Disorders*, 50(6): 721–736.

Salis, C., Murray, L., & Vonk, J. M. J. (2021). Systematic review of subjective memory measures to inform assessing memory limitations after stroke and stroke-related aphasia. *Disability and Rehabilitation*, 43(11): 1488–1506. doi: 10.1080/09638288.2019.1668485

Sohlberg, M. M., Kennedy, M., Avery, J., Coelho, C., Turkstra, L., Ylvisaker, M., & Yorkston, K. (2007). Evidence-based practice for the use of external aids as a memory compensation technique. *Journal of Medical Speech – Language Pathology*, 15(1): xv–li.

Swinburn, K., Porter, G., Howard D. (2023). *The Comprehensive Aphasia Test (CAT)*, 2nd ed. Routledge.

Togher, L., Wiseman-Hakes, C., Douglas, J., Stergiou-Kita, M., Ponsford, J., Teasell. R., Bayley, M., & Turkstra, L. S. (2014). INCOG recommendations for management of cognition following traumatic brain injury, Part IV: cognitive communication. *Journal of Head Trauma Rehabilitation*, 29(4): 353–368. doi: 10.1097/HTR.0000000000000071

FURTHER READING

Bowen, A., & Lincoln N. B. (2007).Cognitive rehabilitation for spatial neglect following stroke. *Cochrane Database of Systematic*

Reviews, 2: Art. No.: CD003586. doi:10.1002/14651858.CD003586.pub2

Fight for Sight https://www.fightforsight.org.uk/about-the-eye/a-z-eye-conditions/hemianopia

Lassaletta, A. (2020). *The Invisible Brain Injury.* Routledge Press.

https://www.rcslt.org/members/clinical-guidance/long-covid/long-covid-guidance/#section-10

Sacks, O. (1985). *The Man Who Mistook His Wife for a Hat.* Picador Press.

Tactus https://tactustherapy.com/app/vat

Villard, S., & Kiran, S. (2016). To what extent does attention underlie language in aphasia? *Aphasiology,* 31(10): 11226–1245.

Zakarias, L., Keresztes, A., Marton, K., & Wartenburger, I. (2016). Positive effects of a computerised working memory and executive function training on sentence comprehension in aphasia. *Neuropsychological Rehabilitation,* 28(3): 369–386. doi: 10.1080/09602011.2016.1159579

Chapter 6

CLINICAL DIAGNOSIS: ASSOCIATED COMMUNICATION DISORDERS

When you are working with people with aphasia, you may need to take into account speech production problems that are related to muscle weakness (dysarthria) or control (apraxia of speech (AoS)). Assessment of someone's communication after e.g. a stroke or ABI should take these into account alongside the aphasia. Therapy can often incorporate exercises that are helpful for both.

56 APRAXIA OF SPEECH (AoS)

Verbal apraxia or apraxia of speech usually occurs alongside aphasia, but there is no clear agreement as to exactly what it is. It is possible to view it as a separate disorder; a problem with planning or programming the muscle movements needed to articulate speech, so a motor speech disorder, rather than a language disorder. However, you are unlikely to see someone who presents with only AoS; a rare case of severe AoS without any aphasia has been reported (Pracar et al. 2023). Many of the features of aphasic spoken word production difficulties and AoS are shared (e.g. difficulties initiating speech, slowed rate of speech, repeated attempts to correct spoken word errors, audible and visual 'groping' for a word, increased errors as individual words become more complex with increased syllable length, automatic speech more accurate and fluent than propositional speech). So, what one clinician labels as AoS may be seen as aphasic word retrieval difficulties by another, often depending on clinical training. It matters because it will not be enough for a client to only target motor speech production and not any underlying language difficulties.

ASSESSMENT:

Make sure you have assessed someone's auditory and written comprehension skills and, when you look at their speech production, that you assess naming, repetition and reading aloud; look for what their aphasia involves and how that is affecting speech production before assuming AoS. Assessment of suspected AoS should note the following key characteristics as being most useful for diagnosis, looking at these in someone's speech in conversation, repetition and automatic speech (Wambaugh et al. 2006):

- Speech rate slow due to some sounds being lengthened (vowels and/or syllables)
- Speech rate slow due to lengthy hesitations between sounds/words (sometimes an extra schwa sound added in the pause)
- Speech sounds distorted (vowels and consonants)
- Speech sounds substituted
- Speech sound errors consistent in type (omission, distortion, substitution)
- Abnormal prosody: e.g. equal stress on all syllables in an utterance.

The most well-known standardised assessment is the *Apraxia Battery for Adults* (ABA) (Dabul 2000). This has subtests, including looking at someone's diadochokinetic rate, repeating words of increasing length, speech samples, limb and oral apraxia (see Assessment Appendix 4).

TREATMENT

Many treatments of AoS focus on how the speech articulators are moving, and use the principles of motor learning, e.g. taking into account how much practice is done, what kind of feedback there is. Techniques that have been shown to facilitate speech production involve the therapist modelling sounds, immediate and delayed repetition and oral reading (face-to-face or computerised therapy). Other treatments include ultrasound, used as visual biofeedback, providing images of the shape and positioning of the tongue to someone as they attempt speech, for example, and melodic intonation therapy (MIT). MIT therapy includes musical intonation patterns and hand tapping alongside speech attempts. There are apps, e.g. Tactus and Speech Sounds on Cue, that provide repeated practice of sounds and words (plus corresponding pictures and written words). A key beneficial feature for people with aphasia and AoS is being able to hear a sound and have articulatory cueing via a video of someone speaking. Therapy approaches can combine treatment of both the aphasia and AoS; your choice of which words and functional phrases (content and length) can take both into account (see links in Further Reading).

OTHER APRAXIAS

Other apraxias are relevant to your work with people with aphasia. **Oral apraxia** may occur alongside AoS, or not. It involves being unable to perform voluntary muscle movements in the oral tract, with intact sensory motor functions (someone may not be able to lick their lips or smile to command but can lick an ice-cream and smile at a friend). Remember to assess whether someone understands the spoken or written commands to perform a movement; their ability to lick their lips, for example, may be the result of a comprehension deficit rather than/as well as oral apraxia. **Limb apraxia** affects around 30 per cent of people after a stroke. It prevents someone from being able to use gesture easily instead of spontaneous speech (including being able to point at what they want).

ASSESSMENT

There is an apraxia screening in the *Boston Diagnostic Aphasia Examination* (see Assessment Appendix 4). There are screening as well as diagnostic tests that identify limb apraxia in stroke patients (see Further Reading).

TREATMENT

Rehabilitation uses behavioural therapies (either restorative or compensatory) and can provide treatment for both someone's aphasia and apraxia. Restorative therapy might be semantic association exercises, e.g. what does this tool do, how do we use it; along with appropriate gesture training (see Point 81). Compensatory interventions focus on training with strategies and support from conversation partners. You may work alongside occupational therapists and physiotherapists in assessing and treating oral and limb apraxias.

57 DYSARTHRIA

Dysarthria is a motor speech disorder, involving slower and weaker movements of the muscles needed to produce both speech and voice. It is caused by damage to the central or peripheral nervous system, and you are likely to be treating clients with aphasia and dysarthria (around 25 per cent of people after a stroke or acquired brain injury (ABI) present with both) (Mitchell et al. 2018). Dysarthria can be divided into seven types or sub-categories:

- **Unilateral Upper Motor Neuron:** This dysarthria is caused by focal lesions after a stroke, traumatic brain injury (TBI), tumour and when the lesion is in the left hemisphere, occurs alongside aphasia. When in the right hemisphere, it occurs alongside cognitive deficits (see chapter 5 cognitive and right hemisphere below).
- **Flaccid:** A TBI, tumour or brain stem stroke may damage cranial or spinal nerves important for speech production, e.g. weak and imprecise tongue movements from damage to the hypoglossal cranial nerve (XII).
- **Spastic:** A brainstem stroke or tumour, TBI, cerebral anoxia or infection can cause bilateral damage to upper motor

neurons leading to weak, slow, imprecise/tight movements of the lips, tongue or vocal cords.

- **Ataxic:** A stroke, brain tumour or TBI as well as degenerative disease can all cause damage to the cerebellum, which impairs coordination of the timing, speed, direction and strength of muscle movements.
- **Mixed:** Mixed dysarthria is mainly seen in degenerative conditions such as multiple sclerosis (MS), motor neuron disease (MND) but is also seen after a brainstem stroke, multiple strokes, TBI or tumour.
- **Hypokinetic:** Hypokinetic dysarthria is caused by dysfunction of the extrapyramidal system, specifically the basal ganglia, e.g. Parkinson's disease or viral encephalitis. It normally affects all aspects of speech production (breathing, voice production, resonance, articulation and prosody).
- **Hyperkinetic:** Hyperkinetic dysarthria is also a result of damage to the extrapyramidal system which can be caused by stroke, tumour, degenerative, inflammatory causes or brain injury. Speech difficulties result from the sudden, brief, involuntary muscle movements (myoclonus) that disturb the rate and rhythm of speech production, e.g. Tourette's syndrome, Huntington's disease.

Alongside dysarthria, people with degenerative neurological conditions may present with language comprehension and production difficulties, e.g. word retrieval difficulties (Cuoco et al. 2021) and cognitive difficulties. These combine to have a negative impact on someone's ability to engage in conversation, so any SLT provision needs to assess and treat all these deficits.

ASSESSMENT

This may involve informal, perceptual clinical assessment and instrumental assessment (if appropriate or available). Assessment may include an examination of oral motor movements, of voice production via informal and/or formal rating scales and tools (see Assessments in Further Reading below).

TREATMENT

Treatment aims to help someone with dysarthria to communicate within the limitations of the neurological condition that has caused the dysarthria (particularly when it is a degenerative condition) and within the framework of the International Classification of Functioning, Disability and Health (ICF). Treatments can be **behavioural**; teaching new skills, compensating for areas of speech production that are impaired. They can include establishing the best posture someone can achieve, education and practice in breath support for voice and speech production, exercises for muscle strengthening and contrastive exercises for intonation and speech rate control. The Lee Silverman Voice Treatment (LSVT®) (see Further Reading) is an intensive treatment with the goal of producing a consistently loud enough voice in conversation including high vocal effort and recalibration of an appropriate level of loudness; the cognitive ability to calibrate volume is impaired in people with several neurological disorders. LSVT® has been shown to improve the speech, voice and communication of people with Parkinson's disease and hypokinetic dysarthria and ataxic dysarthria (e.g. after a stroke). **Compensatory** therapy includes augmentative and alternative communication (AAC) – both low technology and mid/high technology aids (see Point 81,– strategies such as spelling words out loud, using writing or gesture alongside speech and using pacing techniques to slow rate. **Functional** interventions include education about dysarthria, giving advice about ensuring the environment is more helpful, (reducing noise, ensuring the listener is engaged and face-to-face communication and lip reading), learning better self-monitoring, strategies to speak in shorter sentences and communication support from friends and family. When you are treating someone who has both aphasia and dysarthria, there will be opportunities to work on issues that span the two impairments. This may involve working on improving someone's ability to engage in therapy, to focus attention, monitor their speech and understand when and how to modify or repair communication attempts.

58 RIGHT HEMISPHERE DISORDERS

Strokes and TBIs are a common cause of damage to the right hemisphere, as well as brain tumours and infections. Right hemisphere lesions lead to cognitive-communication deficits (see Chapter 5) which need to be considered in any assessment and language therapy. Right hemisphere strokes often lead to visual neglect (affecting reading and writing), attention deficit and cognitive difficulties with executive functions such as planning and reasoning, verbal working memory and non-verbal episodic memory and learning, for example.. The right hemisphere has a role in language processing, including in:

- Lexical-semantic processing (understanding idioms, ambiguity, metaphor, humour)
- Language use; discourse and pragmatics (understanding different forms of communication; narrative, conversations and the social use of language; managing ambiguous information, integrating information, establishing the theme of a conversation, monitoring/maintaining relevance of output or being sensitive to the situation or conversation partner's needs; turn-taking, eye-contact, making and understanding facial expressions)
- Prosody (understanding and using intonation, emphasis and emotion in speech).

There are also some rare difficulties associated with right hemisphere lesions, e.g. prosopagnosia, where familiar faces are no longer recognised.

CROSSED APHASIA

For most people, the right hemisphere is non-dominant for language (whether they are right or left-handed). For a small number of people, language functions are dominant in the right hemisphere, and when this is damaged it leads to what is termed 'crossed aphasia'.

REFERENCES

Cuoco, S., Picillo, M., Carotenuto, I., Erro, R., Catricalà, E., Cappa, S., Pellecchia, M. T., & Barone, P. (2021). The language profile in multiple system atrophy: an exploratory study. *Journal of Neural Transmission*, 128(8): 1195–1203.

Dabul B. (2000). *Apraxia Battery for Adults*, 2nd ed. Pro-Ed.

Mitchell, C., Bowen, A., Gittins, M., Vail, A., Conroy, P., Paley, L., Bray, B., & Tyson, S. (2018). Prevalence of aphasia and co-occurrence of dysarthria: the UK Sentinel Stroke National Audit Programme. *Aphasiology*, 32(sup1): 145–146. doi: 10.1080/02687038.2018.1485863b

Pracar, A. L., Ivanova, M. V., Richardson, A., & Dronkers, N. F. (2023). A case of pure apraxia of speech after left hemisphere stroke: behavioural findings and neural correlates. *Frontiers in Neurology*, 14: 1187399. doi: 10.3389/fneur.2023.1187399

Wambaugh, J. L:, Duffy, J., McNeil, M., Robin, D., & Rogers, M. (2006). Treatment guidelines for acquired apraxia of speech: a synthesis and evaluation of the evidence. *Journal of Medical Speech-Language Pathology*, 14(2): xv–xxxiii.

FURTHER REFERENCES

Albert, M. L., Sparks, R. W., & Helm, N. A. (1973). Melodic intonation therapy for aphasia. *Archives of Neurology*, 29: 130–131. doi:10.1001/archneur.1973.00490260074018

Aphasia Software Finder. https://www.aphasiasoftwarefinder.org/search/node?keys=apraxia

Bishop, C. (2004). *Speech Sounds on Cue*. Propella Multimedia Ltd. www.propeller.net https://mmsp.com.au/product/speech-sounds-on-cue-for-iphone-and-ipad

Bloch, S. and Beeke, S. (2021) A better conversations approach for people living with dysarthria. In M. Walshe and N. Miller (Eds.), *Clinical Cases in Dysarthria*. Routledge.

Duffy, J. R. l. (2005). *Motor Speech Disorders: Substrates, Differential Diagnosis, and Management* (2nd ed.). Elsevier Mosby.Duffy, J. (2013). Apraxia of speech. In J. Duffy (Ed.), *Motor Speech Disorders: Substrates, Differential Diagnosis and Management*, 3rd ed. Elsevier Mosby.

Hegde, M. N., & Freed, D. (2011). *Dysarthria: Assessment of Communication Disorders in Adults*. Plural Publishing. (For differential diagnosis and assessment of AoS.)

Helm-Estabrooks N. (2002). Diagnostic and treatment issues of apraxia. *Seminars in Speech and Language,* 23(4): 219–220.

Lee Silverman Voice Treatment (LSVT®) https://www.lsvtglobal.com

McNeil, M. R., Robin, D. A., & Schmidt, R. A. (2009). Apraxia of speech: theory and differential diagnosis. In M. R. McNeil, *Clinical Management of Sensorimotor Speech Disorders,* 2nd ed. (pp. 249–269). Thieme Medical.

Mitchell, C., Bowen, A., Tyson, S., Butterfint, Z., & Conroy, P. (2017). Interventions for dysarthria due to stroke and other adult-acquired, non-progressive brain injury. *Cochrane Database System Review* 1(1): CD002088. doi: 10.1002/14651858 CD002088.pub3

Narayana, S., Franklin, C., Peterson, E., Hunter, E. J., Robin, D. A., Halpern, A., Spielman, J., Fox, P. T., & Ramig, L. O. (2022). Immediate and long-term effects of speech treatment targets and intensive dosage on Parkinson's disease dysphonia and the speech motor network: randomized controlled trial. *Human Brain Mapping,* 43(7): 2328–2347. doi.org/10.1002/hbm.25790

Papathanasiou, I., & Coppens, P. (2002). *Aphasia and Related Neurogenic Communication Disorders.* 3rd ed. Jones and Bartlett Learning. (Useful rules of thumb for distinguishing between apraxia, aphasia and dysarthria.)

Preston, J., & Leaman, M. (2014). Ultrasound visual feedback for acquired apraxia of speech: a case report. *Aphasiology,* 28: 278–295. doi:10.1080/02687038.2013.852901

Ramig, L. O., Halpern, A., Spielman, J., Fox, C., & Freeman, K. (2018). Speech treatment in Parkinson's Disease: randomized controlled trial (RCT). *Movement Disorders,* 33(1): 1777–1791. doi.org/10.1002/mds.27460

Stark, B. C., & Warburton, E. A. (2018). Improved language in chronic aphasia after self-delivered iPad speech therapy. *Neuropsychological Rehabilitation,* 28(5): 818–831.

Stocks, R., Dacakis, G., Phyland, D., & Rose, M. (2009). The effect of smooth speech on the speech production of an individual with ataxic dysarthria. *Brain Injury,* 23(10): 820–829. doi: 10.1080/02699050902997888 (Parts of a treatment provided to people with dysfluency, 'Smooth Speech', which includes delayed auditory feedback and prolonged speech, has been used to treat ataxic dysarthria, hypokinetic dysarthria and AoS.)

Tactus Therapy https://tactustherapy.com/app/apraxia

Varley, R., Cowell, P. E., Dyson, L., Inglis, L., Roper, A., & Whiteside, S. P. (2016). Self-administered computer therapy for apraxia of speech: two-period randomized control trial with crossover. *Stroke*, 47(3), 822–828. doi:10.1161/STROKEAHA.115.011939

Walshe, M. and Miller, N. (Eds.). (2022). *Clinical Cases in Dysarthria*. Routledge.

Wambaugh, J. L. (2021). An expanding apraxia of speech (AoS) treatment evidence base: an update of recent developments, *Aphasiology*, 35(4): 442–461. doi: 10.1080/02687038.2020.1732289

Wambaugh, J. L., Wright, S., Mauszycki, S., Nessler, C., & Bailey, D. (2018). Combined Aphasia and Apraxia of Speech Treatment (CAAST): systematic replications in the development of a novel treatment. *International Journal of Speech-Language Pathology*, 20(2): 247–261. doi:10.1080/17549507.2016.1267262

Whiteside, S. P., Dyson, L., Cowell, P. E., Varley, R. A. (2015). The relationship between apraxia of speech and oral apraxia: association or dissociation? *Archives of Clinical Neuropsychology*, 30(7): 670–682. https://doi.org/10.1093/arclin/acv051

Chapter 7

TREATMENTS

59 BRAIN STIMULATION

Non-invasive brain stimulation (NIBS) may increase language recovery following stroke by changing brain function and promoting neuroplasticity. This could add to spontaneous recovery and complement the SLT given for the aphasia. However, these promising results have been shown in clinical trials but have not yet been approved for use in aphasia therapy clinics. Transcranial magnetic stimulation (TMS) and rTMS (repetitive transcranial magnetic stimulation) involve using coils of wires passed through the scalp that send magnetic pulses to excite neurons in specific parts of the hemisphere where there has been damage. This may help the brain to 'reorganise' signals around the lesion(s) or suppress them in the hemisphere opposite the lesion(s). It has shown positive results for people with anomia and it is thought that it reduces the abnormally high activation in the undamaged (right) hemisphere, which results in the reactivation of key language areas in the damaged left hemisphere. Functional magnetic resonance imaging (fMRI) (see Point 9) showed this reactivation and there was significant improvement in naming and in functional speech, beyond treatment. The other brain stimulation technique that has been applied to people with aphasia with positive results (alongside regular SLT for anomia) is transcranial direct current stimulation (tDCS), where weak electrical currents are applied directly to the head.

60 MEDICATION

Medication to treat aphasia following a stroke or neurodegenerative disease (pharmacotherapy) may have several benefits, including priming the brain for therapy, augmenting the gains of therapy and speeding up recovery. It aims to have an impact on the neurotransmitter systems increasing neuroplasticity after stroke. More research is needed to tell us more about the impact on communication deficits.

While brain stimulation and pharmacotherapy are promising developments, with the potential to support recovery, the treatment with the best evidence for producing positive changes in communication for someone with aphasia remains speech and language therapy.

FURTHER READING

Berthier, M., & Davila, G. (2015). *Pharmacology and Aphasia*. Routledge.

Cappa, S. F. (2011). The neural basis of aphasia rehabilitation: evidence from neuroimaging and neurostimulation. *Neuropsychological Rehabilitation,* 21(5): 742–754. https://doi.org/10.1080/09602011.2011.614724

Dávila, G., & Berthier, M. L. (2024). Are pharmacotherapeutics effective for treating aphasia? *Expert Review of Neurotherapeutics*, 24(3): 267–271. https://doi.org/10.1080/14737175.2024.2313557

Miniussi, C., Cappa,, S. F., Cohen, L. G., Floel A, Fregni F, Nitsche, M.A., Oliveri, M., Pascual-Leone, A., Paulus, W., Priori, A., & Walsh, V. (2008). Efficacy of repetitive transcranial magnetic stimulation/transcranial direct current stimulation in cognitive neurorehabilitation. *Brain Stimulation*, 1(4): 326–336.

Seniów, J., Waldowski, K., Leśniak, M, Iwański, S., Czepiel, W., & Członkowska, A. (2013). Transcranial magnetic stimulation comb.ined with speech and language training in early aphasia rehabilitation: a randomized double-blind controlled pilot study. *Topics in Stroke Rehabilitation*, 20(3): 250–261. https://doi.org/10.1310/tsr2003-250

Chapter 8

THE THERAPIST, THE THERAPEUTIC RELATIONSHIP AND DIFFERENT ROLES

61 WHAT DO YOU NEED TO BE?

What do you need to be to do your job as an aphasia therapist? A good place to start is to ask what people with aphasia need you to be. Adults with acquired communication disorders reported wanting their clinician to be many things, including knowledgeable, confident, understanding, practical and inspiring, and to offer them comfort as well as empowering them (Fourie 2009). This list is both inspiring and demanding. You may be at the beginning of your career and in the process of becoming a therapist. Be reassured that even after decades working as an aphasia therapist, you continue to learn and improve. To be a good enough therapist, you continue to learn about aphasia, about aphasia therapy, about how to provide therapy in the most useful way for your clients. It is a good idea not to be too confident about what you do. That frisson of anticipation before a session keeps you on your toes. Developing as a clinician should include taking time to reflect on your therapy sessions, on your own and in discussion with colleagues and a clinical supervisor. Acknowledge what went well and what did not go so well. Don't hesitate to critique your work, it will make you a better therapist and lead to more justifiable confidence in what you do.

62 THE THERAPEUTIC RELATIONSHIP

The relationship between the client and the therapist is central to the success of any therapy. So, part of our work is to build this essential working relationship with each client. As a students you observe the different styles of the therapists you work with and are influenced by that. You can continue to learn from observing the different ways of engaging and interacting with clients and their families. It can be helpful to reflect on the times you were the client and what you appreciated about the relationship with your health care provider/therapist.

63 A SUPPORTIVE ENVIRONMENT

Central to the therapeutic relationship and the therapy setting is providing an environment that is supportive, where there is privacy and confidentiality. Having and showing interest in your client as a person, speaking to them as an autonomous adult worthy of respect, 'I know that you know …' (Kagan 1995) not interrupting or talking over them. Communication is about connecting with other people to share information, emotions and thoughts. In a therapy session, we offer people with aphasia structured therapy practice, strategies, skills and opportunities to connect. People with aphasia are experiencing failure – in their ability to communicate and make themselves understood. This can lead to the person with aphasia avoiding communicating, and/or other people not engaging in conversation with them. Often when someone with aphasia tries to communicate, the attempts are full of errors and are unsuccessful. An essential part of your interaction in therapy is when you acknowledge the difficulties that the aphasia brings and show that conversation is a joint endeavour. Acknowledge success and strengths as well as slow progress and failures. By being someone with whom communication is possible, we build a relationship in which someone with aphasia can be as they are, hopefully with less embarrassment and frustration.

64 INTERACTIONS

How we interact with our clients during treatment can influence the therapeutic relationship and someone's willingness to engage with therapy. Providing language therapy means that you often control the interactions, sometimes with a particular structure (request–response–evaluation) which will highlight errors, but which is necessary for many therapy tasks. It is important to be aware of what you say and the language you use. Be aware of how you correct someone's errors. There is a time to model the correct form of a word or sentence, a time to cue words. When working on more constrained tasks, e.g. sentence production, where you are working on accuracy of word order/semantic roles so that it matters greatly if there are errors, there will be more useful ways to comment on errors than others. Firstly, focus on what was correct. 'OK, you got this bit'. Make the error an issue, rather than their mistake; 'this bit can be tricky' or 'oh, that's often the difficult bit in a sentence'. If appropriate to that client and their personality, use humour carefully. Try a little and see how they react. Responses can be supportive, using non-committal nods and 'mmm' to encourage and keep up the connection between the people in the interaction.

In conversation, it is appropriate to focus on how someone with aphasia gets their message across. Look at how you cue more subtly, ask for more information or repeat the partial information given, get them back on track to continue after checking/clarifying that you have understood: 'I understood that' or 'you made that clear' ('with your gesture/the letters you wrote, along with your speech'). Be specific about what was helpful in getting the message across so the focus is on the goal of clear messages, however they are achieved, via any modality and whether or not there are errors. Interactions should be between people, so check how much of the session is taken up with you doing the talking. Do you control who talks and when, and what the topics of conversation are and when they change (Simmons-Mackie & Damico 2011)?

65 MAKE CONNECTIONS

The listening we do is not only to find out more about someone's aphasia but to build the therapeutic relationship and to connect with our client and their family. When we listen, we discover who these people are, what interests and lives they have and what they talk about. We can then relate to the information we have learned so that conversations are more meaningful. To make sure we have interactions that are not centred around the therapy task and more like everyday communication, it is important to build this rapport in the session by valuing the 'small talk'; the conversations about the weather, family news, upcoming shared times of the year (spring in the air, Christmas) as well as the larger stories they may wish to tell and be listened to telling. Look for where your client takes the lead in the conversation, initiates topics and talks more.

66 BRING YOURSELF TO THE THERAPY SESSION

Some aphasia therapy is delivered via computer software, but essentially it involves human beings and human connection, and we are not robots. So, you will inevitably bring yourself to the therapy sessions, which is part of building a relationship with your client and their families. When we start working as SLTs, there is usually an imbalance between how much the client reveals about themselves and how much we might say about ourselves. This may be appropriate, but be careful not to hide behind your role. We may hide behind our role as SLT because we think we have to present ourselves as an all-knowing clinician rather than a person who has useful skills to offer.

It is important that while being the SLT you are also yourself, that you are 'genuine' (as with any client-centred therapy) (Rogers 1961). An eminent psychiatrist, Irvin Yalom (2010), suggests tips for new therapists, which are interesting and helpful for aphasia therapists to read. They include letting the client matter to you (not hiding behind a role), creating a new therapy for each client (very true; no one with aphasia and no therapy for them is ever completely the same) and (almost) never make decisions for them. We may make suggestions, offer options. Losing your language can disenfranchise you and aphasia therapists should aim to empower our clients (see Point 69).

Finding a way to bring yourself to the therapy session that you feel comfortable with is something you will develop over the years. Discuss it with colleagues and with a clinical supervisor (see Chapter 10, Point 100). It will change as you change, with your knowledge and experience of aphasia and of aphasia therapy and with your personal experiences of relationships, of illness and bereavement. Stay curious. Listen and notice. Be knowledgeable and flexible. Hold the space for communication that is different, difficult. Connect with your client and family appropriately. Alongside the assessment , goal setting and treatment, navigate the difficulties that persist and celebrate the successes together and end the relationship with care.

67 OWN YOUR EXPERTISE

You may not feel like one, but you are likely to be, if not an expert, then the person in the room who is most knowledgeable about aphasia therapy. You are an important part of your client's journey to improving their communication. So, lots of pressure, yes. And always say when you are not sure and find out the information needed and possible answers or solutions. You may be the expert in the multi-disciplinary team (MDT) on a ward or a virtual MDT that meets online. Colleagues will look to you to understand and explain the communication difficulties the person with aphasia has, to advise them on the most successful ways to communicate and perhaps provide training about aphasia, including teaching strategies to have better conversations. It can seem obvious to an SLT to use writing alongside speech when having a conversation with someone with aphasia, but it can be a revelation to other health care professionals. So, start with the basics. Have confidence in your knowledge, the importance of those basics and in promoting them.

You may be called to be an expert witness, providing evidence to help with a legal process in court. As an aphasia therapist, you are most likely to be involved in a personal injury case, or in a medical negligence claim where someone has a brain injury and seeks compensation. You provide a written report outlining the assessment of the impact of the brain injury on someone's communication and the consequences for their quality of life, including being able to work and participate in social activities; you suggest how much therapy may be needed and what that therapy may achieve (see Point 19). Depending on your work environment, you may be part of a team that is involved in a legal case and would have the support of colleagues. Your professional organisation (in the UK, the RCSLT)[1] can provide support to members, including some legal advice in situations where you are required to give evidence to a court about a client.

68 SHARE EXPERTISE

Initially, when the aphasia is new for someone, people will usually rely on your expertise to explain aphasia and suggest therapy. Recognise the wealth of what you know and its limitations. You understand the concepts, the complexities in the abstract. The person with aphasia has knowledge and experience that comes from living with aphasia. Their family also understand aphasia it in a way that you cannot. Acknowledging the different types of knowledge and working to combine them is an important part of aphasia therapy. Take a 'team' approach, with each person bringing their expertise to every stage of aphasia therapy. Working collaboratively on goal setting is an example of this. You may suggest options that are clinically realistic, but the decisions are made by the client and family and this joint working results in better outcomes (Rose, Rosewilliam & Soundy 2017). Aphasia therapists benefit from seeing themselves not as 'the first violinists, but conductors of a harmonious orchestra' (Basso & Macis 2011).

69 ADVOCATE

One situation where our role may be an advocate for our client with aphasia is in the assessment and management of decision-making and mental capacity issues. The Mental Capacity Act became law in the UK in 2005 to protect and empower people who may lack the capacity or are at risk of compromised capacity. According to this law, someone lacks capacity if, 'at the time, he is unable to make a decision for himself because of an impairment of, or a disturbance in the functioning of, the mind or brain' (Johnston & Liddle 2005) The mental capacity legislation varies across the UK, but all mental capacity assessments should consider if a person can:

- Understand information that is relevant to the decision
- Retain this information
- Use or weigh this information to make a decision
- Communicate the decision.

Because we have detailed knowledge of someone's communication abilities, we can advocate for them to contribute to best interest meetings, for example. Sometimes it may have been assumed that they lack the capacity to make their own choices and decisions. We may be in the role of facilitating another health care professional to carry out a capacity assessment where supported conversation techniques can enable someone with aphasia to understand complex issues and indicate choices.

This is very much the work we normally do using supported conversation to enable people to understand information and get their message across. See the useful resource from the Aphasia Centre (Kagan, Shumway & MacDonald 2020). It is useful to read case studies and talk to other clinicians about doing the work, and the format it takes, particularly in report writing. The opinion of the SLT may be that someone can access the meaning of the message if their conversation is supported; information is given in several formats (spoken, written, drawings or gestures). Questions can be closed (that need only a yes or no answer, which can be given via speech or gesture or by pointing to a written word or symbol). Repeating questions and information can make a significant difference to people with aphasia. A visual format such as Talking Mats (Murphy, Cameron & Boa 2013)[2] is often essential in these assessments. Similarly, someone with aphasia who appears unable to communicate their decision because they lack sufficient speech, may be able to use writing, pointing to written words and/or pictures or gestures to do so (see also Chapter 10, Point 94).

NOTES

1 Royal College of Speech & Language Therapists https://www.rcslt.org
2 https://www.talkingmats.com

REFERENCES

Basso, A., & Macis, M. (2011). Therapy efficacy in chronic aphasia. *Behavioural Neurology*, 24(4): 317–325. doi: 10.3233/BEN-2011-0342

Ferguson, A., & Armstrong, E. (2004). Reflections on speech-language therapists' talk: implications for clinical practice and education. *International Journal of Language and Communication*, 39(4): 469–477.

Fourie, R. J. (2009). A qualitative study of the therapeutic relationship in speech and language therapy: perspectives of adults with acquired communication and swallowing disorders. *International Journal of Language & Communication Disorders*, 44(6): 979–999.

Johnston, C., & Liddle, J. (2007). The Mental Capacity Act 2005: a new framework for healthcare decision making. *Journal of Medical Ethics*. 33(2): 94–97. doi: 10.1136/jme.2006.016972.

Kagan, A. (1995). Revealing the competence of aphasic adults through conversation: a challenge to health professionals. *Topics in Stroke Rehabilitation*, 2(1): 15–28.

Kagan, A., Shumway, E., & MacDonald, S. (2020). Assumptions about decision-making capacity and aphasia: ethical implications and impact. *Seminars in Speech and Language*, 41(3): 221–231. https://aphasia-institute.s3.amazonaws.com/uploads/2022/10/Kagan-Shumway-MacDonald_CAC21vFF_.pdf

Murphy, J., Cameron, L., & Boa, S. (2013). *Talking Mats: A Resource to Enhance Communication.* 2nd ed.). Available at: https://www.talkingmats.com and https://www.rcslt.org/wp-content/uploads/2020/12/TM-20201008-TM-RCSLT-guidance-text.pdf

Rogers, C. (1961). *On Becoming a Person: A Therapist's View of Psychotherapy.* Constable.

Rose, A., Rosewilliam, S., & Soundy, A. (2017). Shared decision-making in goal setting in rehabilitation settings: a systematic review. *Patient Education and Counselling,* 100(1): 65–75.

Simmons-Mackie, N., & Damico, J. (2011). Exploring clinical interaction in speech-language therapy: narrative, discourse and relationships. In R. J. Fourie (Ed.), *Therapeutic Processes for Communication Disorders* (pp. 35–52). Psychology Press.

Yalom, I. (2010). *The Gift of Therapy: An Open Letter to a New Generation of Therapists and Their Patients.* Piatkus.

FURTHER READING

Hale, S. (2003). *The Man Who Lost His Language.* Penguin Books. (See Chapter 13 for an example of a working relationship.)

Martin, N., Thompson, C. K., & Worrall, L. (2008). *Aphasia Rehabilitation: The Impairment and its Consequences.* Plural Publishing.

Volkmer, A. (2016). *Dealing with Capacity and Other Legal Issues with Adults with Acquired Neurological Conditions: A Resource for SLTs.* J&R Press.

Chapter 9

THERAPY

70 WHAT IS IT?

The brain stimulation and pharmacotherapy treatments outlined in Chapter 7 may become more widely used in the future. Currently, the treatment with the best evidence for producing positive changes in communication for someone with aphasia remains behavioural therapy provided by speech and language therapists. Behavioural therapy assumes that despite the brain lesions, neural plasticity gives people with aphasia the potential to improve their language and communication (as long as they receive the appropriate amount and type of treatment). The different approaches to aphasia suggest different mechanisms or ways through which therapy achieves this improved communication. If aphasia is due to impaired access to language, then therapy can restore this access and reconnect the language processes (impairment-based treatments). If the damaged language processes cannot be retrained, therapy focuses on using the remaining language skills to compensate and learn to use as strategies (compensatory treatments).

71 FIRST KEY STEPS

Assessment will have given you an initial understanding of a client's aphasia and shown you how they are able or trying to communicate, either with or beyond speech. Early therapy includes providing information about aphasia to your client and the people around them, encouraging all communication and trialling different ways to communicate. Start with what they can do, use the modality they are more successful using and use this to negotiate some initial goals with them to inform therapy targets.

How therapy is chosen and how it is delivered is key to its success. So, make sure you make time to consider what approach you will take and to plan and prepare therapy. Think about the targets you are working on in therapy, what tasks you choose and why you think this therapy will improve a language skill(s), and/or learning strategies, for everyday communication.

Your session plan should clearly describe what the task is, what you are aiming for your client to do, what cues you will use, how you will measure responses (in the sessions, with audio/video recordings and contemporaneous notes) and how you will increase or decrease the difficulty of the task. Keep written records, chart progress and changes, e.g. in cues needed, any generalisation. Make your plan clear enough for another clinician to pick it up and use it to carry out the session. Discuss the therapy plan with your client and be ready to explain why you are presenting these picture matching tasks or asking them to practise this writing app. Plan how many sessions you will work on a treatment in advance, talk to your client about this as part of discussing the end of therapy.

Plan how you will evaluate the success or otherwise of the treatment and measure any progress made (see Further Reading for more information on baseline measurements and evaluating therapy (Lum 2002)). Build up your set of resources, including large enough sets of pictures to use some in treatment and some to evaluate the treatment.

Be flexible; continually check what you are doing, why, what effect it is having and be prepared to change course. You adapt therapy in the light of what you learn about the underlying language deficits and your client's response to treatment.

Take time to go over what happened in that treatment block to build an understanding of why one technique or strategy might have brought about improvements, and another did not. This will build your knowledge and expertise in promoting positive change in a client's language to meet their communication goals.

72 DOES IT WORK?

There is a lot of evidence that aphasia therapy results in more improvement in someone's language abilities than spontaneous recovery does, both at the acute and the chronic stage of aphasia (Yamaji & Maeshima 2022). It improves the comprehension and production of language, e.g. speech, reading, writing and everyday communication after stroke and when the aphasia is due to progressive forms of brain damage (Simmons-Mackie et al. 2017), compared with no therapy (Brady et al. 2016). Neuroimaging studies, during and after treatment, show changes in brain activation with improved language functioning following various therapies (Heath et al. 2022). Impairment-based therapies, including semantic and phonological therapies, can improve auditory comprehension, reading, writing, single word and sentence production (Basso, Capitani & Vignolo 1979) and functional communication, including speech in conversation. Other successful treatments include computer-based therapy, training of communication partners and teaching multimodal strategies (total communication). M-MAT (Rose 2013) is more effective than the 'usual care' of much aphasia therapy provision (either no therapy or less than one hour a week). Intensive programmes (e.g. Leff et al. 2021) providing around 30 hours of therapy for 5 days a week over a 3-week period led to gains on both impairment-based and functional measures of language.

Knowing that there is evidence to show that therapy has a measurable positive change on someone's ability to communicate effectively is important in our understanding of what we can aim to achieve with therapy and our confidence in what we do. Of course, therapy does not always 'work' for every client. If someone's goal is to 'get back to normal' you will need to explore what 'normal' looks like for them. Education about aphasia needs to include the long-lasting difficulties that are the nature of the disorder; even with recovery there are likely to be continuing issues, some significant in terms of the impact on someone's life and some only residual problems. Part of therapy is encouraging your client (and their family) to broaden their understanding of what 'getting better' means. The discussion about this begins when you look at goals, being explicit as to the uncertain results of any therapy, and is continued during treatment, with your monitoring and evaluation of the effectiveness of therapy and any improvements that are meeting these goals and sharing this information with them. Hopefully, one goal you will have introduced is adapting in some way to the aphasia and the changes in communication (see Points 89 and 90).

This links to discharge from therapy; because someone can benefit from therapy over many years, deciding what will work, what that means and when to stop is a careful process of discussion about goals, measuring change, seeing therapy input as part of what is useful for them at that point in managing the aphasia.

For therapy to work, the client and their family have to want therapy. They need to be motivated to attend sessions and do the work, with a commitment to regular home practice of therapy tasks and/or communication strategies essential for change and improvement. When therapy doesn't seem to work and there is a lack of progress, you need to consider many possibilities. Is the client not doing the work because there is a lack of confidence or motivation? Is there disappointment at the lack of hoped-for progress? Is there enough understanding of the nature of aphasia and of rehabilitation on the part of the client and the family? Are there other factors in their lives that prevent regular attendance and home practice?

> Mr. Smith's daughters had referred him to SLT, hoping that it could help their elderly parents with the difficult situation they had been in since their father's stroke and the significant aphasia that followed. The couple barely

looked at each other, spoke at the same time (his speech was mainly unintelligible jargon) and exhibited great irritation with each other (eye-rolling, sighing, shaking fists). The first goal of SLT was to establish listening, turn-taking and some eye contact; essential for any conversation. Mrs. Smith had given up listening because Mr. Smith's speech was unintelligible. Mr. Smith had become frustrated and angry because, as far as he was concerned, there was nothing wrong with his speech, and Mrs. Smith was just not listening. Therapy involved some assessment to find out what Mr. Smith's comprehension of spoken words and reading was like and what he could do to get any part of his message across. It then focused on Total Communication; with Mr. Smith learning to use a combination of writing, drawing and gesture, alongside his vocalisations and speech attempts in structured practice and conversation and Mrs. Smith learning to use the partial information he gave using these strategies and combine them to try and understand the message. To build collaboration, therapy highlighted that the conversation was a shared responsibility; Mr. Smith using strategies, Mrs. Smith listening or watching and building on the message, checking to see if the message was understood correctly by using the strategies herself. Mr. Smith became a better communicator using gesture. Mrs. Smith tried but struggled to understand his gestures. It became apparent that not only did Mr. Smith have aphasia, but Mrs. Smith had cognitive difficulties, too, which was making it difficult for her to learn to communicate in different ways and to be flexible. There were limits to what was possible to achieve in terms of communication success for them, but the collaboration between the couple did lessen the levels of anger and aggression, at least in the therapy sessions. Mr. Smith learnt that his speech was not as effective as he thought, and while he did not want to pursue therapy for his underlying language difficulties, he went on to use Total Communication strategies with his daughters.

73 HOW MUCH AND FOR HOW LONG?

Improvement in language and communication functioning does not generally happen suddenly after a small amount of therapy; progress is usually slow and incremental. While it is still not fully established how much therapy is needed to be effective, neuroplasticity principles suggest that more intensive therapy leads to more recovery and the evidence is clear that the amount of treatment provided is a crucial factor in the achievement of measurable gains in language and communication skills. Intensity or dose of therapy refers to the length of therapy provision, the hours of therapy per week and the total number of hours of therapy provided.

The Cochrane Review (Brady et al. 2016) found that people with aphasia who received therapy at high intensity/high dose, or over a long period of time, had significant improvements in their everyday communication skills, compared with those who received a lower intensity/lower dose of therapy. High intensity in this review means up to 15 hours per week, and long period means 6–9 months rather than 10–12 weeks. NICE guidelines[1] state that rehabilitation for communication difficulties after a stroke should involve treatments of at least 45 mins per day for at least 5 days per week. In one example of an intensive comprehensive aphasia programme (Leff et al. 2021) therapy was provided over a 3-week period, 5 days a week and averaged 6 hours of therapy per day. Bhogal et al. (2003) found a significant positive effect of treatment after 8.8 hours of therapy per week for 11.2 weeks with improved outcomes of speech and language for stroke patients with aphasia. Treatments of around 2 hours per week for 22.9 weeks did not produce the same improvements. On average, there were positive effects after a total of 98.4 hours of therapy, but not after 43.6 hours of therapy. The key finding from this research for clinicians is that a very low dose of therapy may not be effective or may be the equivalent of no therapy at all.

Where there is an option for intensive therapy, it is important to look at each individual client and consider whether they can tolerate such a programme. High-intensity and high-dose interventions may not be acceptable to everyone. There may be mobility or cognitive difficulties and attending sessions in clinic can be a tiring process, there are financial implications, issues of transport, mobility and time commitment (NB see Point 85 for online options). For those that could benefit from an intensive programme, look at what your service could provide, learning from current models which vary in what intensity means (Monnelly, Marshall & Cruice 2021) or at the intensive therapy programmes that might be available for your client. Some intensive programmes in the UK are in clinics attached to universities, sometimes with funding from independent grants, e.g. the Tavistock Aphasia Centre at the University of Newcastle, UK; the ICAP at Queen's Square (Leff et al. 2021) and others (Molino, Egan & Kuschmann 2024).

Remember that dosage is about the total amount of therapy; most importantly, the amount of learning, practice and repetition that the client does in the session. While you may not be able to provide intensive treatment programmes, you should endeavour to provide sufficient dosage and duration of treatment to your client with aphasia. Whatever therapy you are providing, ensure that you work with larger sets of words for practice and that your client practises more words per hour (Thomas et al. 2020).

74 LIMITS ON PROVISION

Unfortunately, there is often an enormous disparity between what the evidence is for how much dosage and intensity is needed to provide beneficial therapy and what we are able to provide. Speech and language therapy provision for many people with aphasia is widely restricted, so that the intensity and dose is much lower than is needed to be effective. In 2018, the median amount of therapy received by people living at home after a stroke in the UK was 6.3 hours in 3 months. On average, one 60-minute session was received every 2 weeks (Palmer, Witts & Chater 2018). Lack of provision may be due to long waiting lists, a shortage of therapists, prioritising dysphagia work or decisions of local managers. Whatever the reason why the therapy service you can offer is limited (see point 24 Ending Therapy), be clear with your client about what you can offer and why. Whatever therapy you can offer, be clear about when therapy will finish from the outset so that everyone knows the timeline for working together.

75 WHICH THERAPY?

While it is not established which therapy or which tasks are the 'best', we operate within current levels of knowledge about therapy techniques and mechanisms of change and therapy procedures. Therapy is likely to include a combination of impairment-based therapy, compensatory therapy and addressing the communication environment, including training of and support from family/friends. We choose one or more therapies to meet the demands of a client's language profile and their goals. Choosing which therapy(s) and how to combine them may depend on how well you know the client and their aphasia and how experienced and comfortable you are with a particular therapy approach and its treatments. At its best, therapy combines the impairment-based and the compensatory-approach to aphasia to treat both the impaired language and the consequences of the aphasia, and involves all of the following approaches:

- rebuilding and restoring language skills
- compensating for lost language skills and learning new ways to communicate
- enabling communication by adapting the environment.

They all aim to change and/or remove the negative impact that aphasia has on someone's ability to engage in their life, understanding aphasia as affecting activities, social connections and participation, work and quality of life. All have been shown to improve the communication of people with aphasia. The A-FROM (see Appendix 1) is useful as a framework for planning therapy. It takes into account the language impairments and the consequences of aphasia on the everyday lives of people with aphasia and their families.

76 IMPAIRMENT-BASED TREATMENT – REBUILDING AND RESTORING LANGUAGE SKILLS

The 'Language and related processes' section of the A-FROM correspond to "Impairment" in the ICF and includes talking, understanding, reading and writing. This approach to aphasia starts with an assessment of someone with aphasia using models of language processing (see Chapters 2 and 4 and the language-processing model in Appendix 2). It suggests which language skills and processes are functioning adequately and which are not. It then uses that information to reach a hypothesis as to which of these processes are causing the communication difficulties and suggests what kind of therapy may rebuild the language skills a client needs. The therapy offered is behavioural, and provides the essential, targeted learning and rebuilding or restoring of language skills. Rebuilding is possible because of neuroplasticity, the brain's ability to change its structure and functioning and both learn and recover language skills. Neural networks can be modified by learning: 'neurons that fire together, wire together' (Hebb 1949), if there is sufficient relearning and practice in treatment.

77 REPETITION

The repetition of tasks is required to rebuild the damaged neural networks and restore language skills. This repetition needs to be of sufficient intensity to ensure learning occurs, meaning that there must be a lot of practice of tasks (or strategies) in therapy to see the change looked for. Present that repetitive practice with confidence. It sometimes helps to compare it with working on particular muscles in the gym; people often understand muscle movements and the need for the same exercises to build ability and you can tie your aphasia therapy into this outlook. And just as people carry out exercises at the gym on different machines or in different ways, you can present your therapy tasks in different ways and formats. The amount of repetitive practice needed has an impact on how the therapy sessions are structured; to ensure enough repetition of tasks you must control what happens in much of the session, so that it involves structured learning, repetition and practice (usually with a request-response-evaluation sequence), mainly in one-to-one sessions. Allocate time for practice, plan how many tasks and how many repetitions across the course of the session, aiming to increase them over the therapy. Ask yourself during (and after) the session: How much am I talking, filling any silence? Was the client active in the session or a passive observer? How much practice did they have attempting speech, writing or gesture? The intensity of practice needed creates challenges in terms of resources for therapy (see Points 73 and 85). Moreover, there are key factors about the way we learn that apply to people with and without aphasia. Learning something, then having a break from it and relearning it is a good model, so we can space out the treatment sessions too. A session should always have conversation and connection; the relationship between the client and therapist has an impact on rehabilitation (see Point 62 in Chapter 8). But concentrate on the client's goals and remember that your job is to help them achieve those goals with targeted therapy, so don't be afraid to make the sessions focused and demanding. Any client needs to have chosen to have therapy, it is important that they are motivated, and that they have the ability and commitment to carry out the tasks both in the therapy session and regularly at home together with the work you give them to do outside sessions. What you model in the session is important for their understanding of how to do the practice at home.

78 LEARNING

Learning involves modelling (so providing examples of the word or gesture) and feedback about responses (clarifying whether it was correct or not). One therapy involves cueing hierarchies to facilitate word production.

CUEING HIERARCHIES

Cueing usually starts by providing the smallest amount of information, adding more as needed to help someone retrieve the word. For example, phonological cueing provides information about the target word, often starting with an initial phoneme cue, or the initial phoneme and grapheme (letter), or with the initial syllable, the number of syllables in the word or a word that rhymes with the target. Semantic cueing includes sentence completion (cut with a ___), providing a category (it's a colour) or definition (it's a long, curved, yellow fruit), function/use (you put it on your head) +/− a gesture. Providing a combination of phonological and orthographic cueing therapy is effective not only for treated but also untreated single words and in connected speech (Greenwood et al. 2010). Use written prompts as part of your therapy for spoken word production. Cueing hierarchy work also involves the client doing more repetition of the target words. Part of cueing therapy is to encourage clients to learn what is helpful for them and work on providing their own cues (using writing, gesture or drawing) to take outside the clinic and into everyday conversation.

FEEDBACK

Feedback about whether a response is correct or not may not be important to promoting successful responses (many people with aphasia are aware of their errors already). It can provide encouragement to continue with the task. What you say when giving feedback and encouragement will need to be appropriate to each individual client and you will need to work out what that is. Remember that you are working with a competent adult, often someone older than you, so be thoughtful and cautious as to how you respond (the words you use) until you get to know them better. Establish a rapport, find out what works for them in terms of helpful responses to attempts, successes and errors. Err on the side of caution as to how you respond until you get to know them better and have established what works for them in terms of helpful responses to attempts, successes and errors.

ERRORS

Errorless learning involves shaping the therapy task to eliminate (or reduce) errors. Rather than trying to avoid any errors, you can reduce the production of errors with the cueing hierarchy you use and with therapy tasks that are easier for that person, slowly introducing more difficult items or levels. Encouraging all attempts at communication, and circumlocution as a strategy to get a message across, will lead to errors. There is some evidence that both errorless and errorful therapy produces the same results, both in the session and long-term.

LEARNING WITH APHASIA

People with aphasia are capable of learning. Even when there is a significant language impairment, words can be taught as if they are new to someone. The ability to learn may be affected by aspects of the aphasia and/or cognitive deficits and you may need to treat these alongside or before the language skills (e.g. treating auditory memory skills to improve understanding spoken sentences in tasks and in everyday communication). This treatment often involves repetition tasks of words and sentences that increase in length and complexity.

79 EXAMPLES OF IMPAIRMENT-BASED THERAPIES

Impairment-based therapy includes treatment for word retrieval, sentence processing, reading, writing, auditory processing and discourse. Your assessment may have shown that your client has word retrieval difficulties or anomia. Perhaps no words are produced in speech or writing. Perhaps they 'talk around' a word (circumlocution) finding some semantic information about the word but not the appropriate phonological information: target 'cigarette': 'smote ... message ... outing ... lit ... burning'). Perhaps making several attempts to get the word right (*conduite d'approche*) where phonological errors are made in the attempt to get closer to the target word, e.g. target 'crab': 'cab, scab, crab'. You will see different types of word errors, some may be semantically related to the intended word (e.g. 'sister' instead of wife or 'carving' instead of knife) or phonologically related (these could be another real word, e.g. 'life' instead of 'wife' or a non-word error – a neologism, where less than 50 per cent of the phonemes of the target is produced – e.g. 'ha' for house). Word errors can be words that are unrelated to the target, e.g. 'hat' for wife. The types of spoken word errors suggest impairments at semantic or phonological levels of language processing, or in the connection between these levels of processing. Difficulty accessing semantic information impairs word comprehension and production and people can benefit from semantic therapy that works to improve access to the meaning of a word (e.g. therapy tasks involving practising spoken or written word to picture matching), semantic category judgement (sorting into category, category generation), feature generation, yes/no feature questions or progressive semantic cues.

SEMANTIC FEATURE ANALYSIS (SFA)

SFA (Boyle 2010) aims to improve word retrieval by stimulating the networks of semantic information around a word. The target word is presented and there are structured questions about the features of the word. SFA therapy can be used to improve access to nouns and verbs. When working on verb retrieval, tasks aim to strengthen the association with semantically related nouns, adjectives, etc. You guide the client to generate the semantic features by giving a description, or sentence completion with where or how the verb is typically done, for example. There is some evidence of generalisation to untreated words with SFA therapy.

PHONOLOGICAL COMPONENTS ANALYSIS (PCA)

PCA (Leonard, Rochon & Laird 2008) treatment is designed to improve word retrieval by working on phonology; similar to SFA, it is also based on the theory of spreading activation and aims to strengthen the phonological networks around target words. The client is prompted to name a picture of a target word and guided to tasks that focus on its phonological features. Phonological therapy tasks include repetition, answering questions about the initial phoneme, rhyme judgements and number of syllables. The theory is that providing the semantic or phonological features of a word activates the semantic or phonological representations for that target and strengthens them (e.g. within the semantic system, in the phonological output lexicon and/or between the output lexicon and the semantic system). PCA tasks also involve semantic processing; while focusing on phonology, the semantic aspects of the picture or word are also processed. Often therapy tasks target both the semantic and phonological levels as both are activated when the word form is presented. The form of the word can be spoken or written, so tasks can target the semantic, phonological and orthographic information about the word. Therapy for **writing** includes **Copy and Recall Treatment (CART)** (Ball et al. 2011). Writing single words is relearned by repeated copying and immediate recall. The three steps involve spoken repetition of a target word in response to a picture, copying the written target word three times and writing the word without a model. This therapy can improve a client's use of writing as an alternative to speech in everyday conversations.

VERBS AND SENTENCE PROCESSING

Verbs are essential for sentence production. The semantic information about verbs may include the knowledge of how the verb relates to other words, what the role of each word is in the sentence and how to build the argument structure of a sentence. People with aphasia may have difficulty not only with retrieving the verb but also with assigning the parts or roles the verbs and associated words play in a sentence, in terms of both what each word means in itself and how the sentence is formed overall: seen here in an attempt to describe the composite picture in the Comprehensive Aphasia Test (CAT) (Swinburn 2023): 'fish ... cat ... slipping ... books ... man ... he's ... coffee ... drink ... book'.

VERB NETWORK STRENGTHENING TREATMENT (VNEST)

VNeST (Edmonds, Mammino & Ojeda 2014) works on word retrieval by strengthening the semantic representation of the verb using sentence level tasks, focusing on the verb's relationship to the thematic roles in the sentence and the argument structure. Therapy involves repetitive practice, using different verbs, in a format where there is a subject (who), a verb (is doing) and an object (what). For example, in the sentence, 'Naomi is stroking the dog' the verb 'stroke' is preceded by 'who?' (Naomi) which is followed by 'what?' (the dog). In therapy tasks this structure and the roles each word plays is practised via questions: What is Naomi doing to the dog? Who is stroking the dog? What is Naomi stroking? Tasks can work on finding other nouns that are in the verb's network (What else can you stroke? Who else could stroke the dog?) and other verbs (What else can you do to a dog?). See Webster and Whitworth (2012) to read about single word and sentence level therapies. See the Newcastle University Aphasia Therapy Resources (Webster et al. 2009) for sentence level therapy work; it has therapy material for working on verb retrieval and comprehension and sentence production. It includes work on argument structure, thematic role assignment and mapping.

MAPPING THERAPY

Mapping therapy focuses on syntax processing and restoring the connections between sentence form and meaning. People with aphasia may have syntactic knowledge but difficulties relating that to semantic information, so that word order and thematic roles are impaired. Mapping therapy involves specific discussion about the role of a verb (agent/patient/theme) and where it is in a sentence. Training in a language process may improve the production and/or comprehension of sentences not explicitly practised in therapy (generalisation) by restoring connections between sentence form and meaning.

AUDITORY COMPREHENSION

Auditory comprehension difficulties have a significant effect on everyday communication and on being able to participate in therapy, particularly in the acute stage. People with significant comprehension difficulties often also have significant language production problems ('global aphasia'). Assessment suggests where the deficits are in the auditory processing system; analysing the phonology of words heard (difficulties at this level causing 'word sound deafness'), accessing the phonological input lexicon ('word form deafness') and accessing the semantic system to be able to understand words heard ('word meaning deafness'). Therapy involves phonological and semantic tasks to remediate those levels of processing. Often we use written routes to comprehension to compensate for auditory comprehension deficits and written tasks in therapy, e.g. spoken word to written word matching, and many people with aphasia have more intact reading ability that can aid auditory comprehension. Semantic therapies for comprehension include categorisation tasks, matching words to pictures and definitions and odd one out judgements. Therapy for auditory processing is needed as well as semantic therapy, e.g. minimal pair discrimination or hearing the word in semantic tasks as well as reading it. In terms of managing conversations, people need impairment-based therapy at the sentence and discourse levels. Targeting cognitive skills such as attention, working memory and executive functions is often important.

With the A-FROM areas of Participation in Life Situations and Communication and Language Environment in mind, impairment-based therapy also addresses the impact of aphasia on someone's everyday life in therapy. Treatments with a participation focus on the use of language and communication in real world contexts look beyond word and sentence level to discourse and conversation. The focus is on everyday communication, so using these different ways of communicating in the real world. Narrative and Discourse Intervention in Aphasia (NADIIA)[2] is a therapy that combines a participation and impairment approach, working on narrative and discourse. It targets single word, sentence and discourse levels and the cognitive skills of planning, monitoring, sequencing to improve discussion and dialogue skills in conversation.

LANGUAGE UNDERPINS NARRATIVE IN APHASIA (LUNA)

LUNA (Dipper et al. 2024) uses different treatments, e.g. semantic feature analysis, mapping therapy (Marshall 1995), to work on language at different linguistic levels with the aim of being able to tell personal stories and narrative. Therapy works on increasing the use of words relevant to the client and expanding their vocabulary, increasing the use of sentences and improving the structure of the narrative and the coherence of the story.

CONSTRAINT INDUCED APHASIA THERAPY (CIAT)

CIAT (Pulvermuller et al. 2001) is a communication-based intervention often delivered in groups that may be helpful in improving sentence and narrative level communication. It is an intensive treatment, with massed practice (30 hours treatment in 2 weeks), involving using only speech to communicate, which the therapist shapes to help production.

THINKING FOR SPEAKING

Your clients may have some cognitive deficits alongside the aphasia but they are not intellectually impaired; they have a specific language disorder. Part of the aphasia may involve difficulties with a level of processing where a pre-verbal message is created, leading to an impairment with 'thinking for speaking'¹ (Slobin 1996). This is the stage of language production where the description of events and situations is structured via inner speech (e.g. selecting what to say and what not to say, understanding the importance of perspective), this message is then mapped onto words and sentence structures. It is possible that aphasia can affect thinking for speaking, so this could be an important area to treat. This can include practice in thinking about situations and events and translating that into language. Look at your client's understanding and use of abstract language and verbs, which may require more awareness of propositional structure and perspective (Levelt 1999), mapping therapy, narrative production with composing messages or thinking through the situation and participants.

80 WORDS FOR THERAPY

It is more common for the improvements we see to be item-specific, that is, if someone works on a set of words or phrases or gestures, they improve their understanding and use of those words/phrases/gestures, both in the clinic and in daily life (Herbert et al. 2003). So, it is important for your client to choose a set of words that are relevant to them, frequently used and of everyday importance. Make sure that you include the various categories of words that are needed in conversation; verbs as well as nouns, not forgetting adjectives, adverbs and pronouns. Use a large set of words (between 60 and 120). People are likely to choose many commonly used words, especially words for food and drink, people, places, clothes, nature, gardening and travel. So, you can prepare a set of pictures or written words using words in those categories for initial practice (Palmer, Hughes & Chater 2017).

81 COMPENSATORY THERAPY

While behavioural therapy aims to restore impaired language skills, a functional or pragmatic approach focuses on the impact aphasia has on everyday communication and social interaction.

Therapy focused on the consequences of the aphasia involves adapting to and compensating for the language loss, both making use of whatever language functions remain and learning alternative ways of communicating. A key part of compensatory therapy is **Total Communication.** This encourages the use of any remaining speech as well as learning to bring in alternative, non-verbal means of communicating. This may include writing, drawing, gesture, using communication boards or other AAC (see below). When someone with aphasia and their conversation partners use these as strategies in a conversation, there can be more success nderstanding others and getting their message across. Therapy includes learning about the different modalities as strategies to choose and benefit from and then practising them. Modality charts or symbols are helpful to make the process explicit in an easy-to-understand way. Present the modality chart and review the communication options (e.g. 'There are many ways to communicate. You can speak, gesture, draw, write, or use your communication book'"). A symbol representing a modality (e.g. a pen with letter above it for writing) can be used as a prompt to try writing or as an acknowledgement that this is the strategy being used.

WRITING

Impairment-based treatment of single word writing can improve the accuracy of writing and this can be used as a strategy in everyday conversation. Work on this in PACE activities (see below), supported conversation practice and group therapy. Writing includes using single letters, parts of words, whole words and an important part of compensatory therapy is to encourage any and all responses, including partially correct responses. You may need to convince both the person with aphasia and the conversation partner to accept part of a word and work collaboratively to piece together the clues that any writing, along with any speech, gesture or drawing may give to understand someone's message. Writing produces information that is fixed for long enough for everyone in the conversation to be able to try and work out what it means. Whiteboards are not as helpful here as pen and paper. People with auditory comprehension difficulties may get more from written information; encourage both the person with aphasia and their conversation partner to use writing to communicate, to provide written choices to support decision making.

GESTURE

Many people with aphasia can make an appropriate gesture for the word they cannot say or write, and these gestures can be used as a strategy to help get their message across. Usually these are symbolic gestures, e.g. thumbs up for yes/good, and pantomimes, e.g. using an object like a mug/key. You cannot assume that someone will be able to understand or use gestures, and people with aphasia tend use gestures differently. Your therapy may involve treating these directly to improve the use of recognisable gestures before promoting the use of gestures to support communication (Rose et al. 2013). Gestures can also act as a cue for speech, framing thoughts for language (Kistner, Dipper & Marshall 2018), so therapy for gestures can also improve word retrieval (particularly verbs).

There are a number of different reasons why the ability to use gestures is impaired. A good level of comprehension and cognitive flexibility are needed to understand how gestures can represent words and can be used in conversation as a strategy to compensate for impaired speech production. Physical difficulties, such as reduced use of one hand or arm, also make producing gestures more challenging. It is important for the SLT to use only one hand/arm when modelling gestures so that the physical difficulties are not felt to be the reason for not using gesture. Limb apraxia causes difficulties with the timing and orientation of the movements for a gesture, ideational apraxia impairs the concepts of movement and intent so that people have difficulty understanding how to use an object. Ideomotor apraxia affects the sequence of motor activity.

DRAWING

Using communicative drawing to exchange information or express a thought does not depend on being able to draw well. Like gesture, the language, cognitive and any motor deficits caused by the brain lesion are likely to mean that you will need to do some drawing practice and give some examples and instructions to promote drawing as a means of communicating a message. Many people do not initiate drawing to aid communication without encouragement and models. Many are using a non-dominant hand and need practice with this. Many do not appreciate which details are needed and which are not and need to work on key features of an object and recognising when they omit or distort features. You do need to draw efficiently; know what information is essential to get the message across and what are irrelevant details, correct or change the drawing in response to questions. This work overlaps with impairment-based semantic feature therapy tasks. Drawing involves cognitive and language skills such as organising thoughts, generating ideas and selecting and discarding information. Therapy can work on copying, tracing or matching an object or picture to a drawing, creating drawings that describe situations or drawing another item in response to two drawings, e.g. after being shown a picture of a banana and an orange, draw another fruit. Drawing is useful in Total Communication as it provides a permanent record of someone's communication attempt and one that the people in conversation can interpret together. Drawing is often the least preferred strategy; it can be time-consuming and effortful for many people. For others, it provides an opportunity to take their turn in the conversation and create a message. It is important that this message is acknowledged and responded to (see Point 82). Like gesture, drawing may encourage spoken word production, particularly nouns.

AUGMENTATIVE AND ALTERNATIVE COMMUNICATION (AAC)

Augmentative and alternative communication (AAC) involves strategies and devices that can enhance or replace speech. In addition to strategies such as writing, gesture and drawing, there are AAC devices or aids (low and high technology). Low technology aids include alphabet charts (useful to point to letters to spell out words), communication boards (point to pictures or written words), rating scales (point to faces, for example, to indicate emotional state), communication books and personalised communication passports (with key written words and phrases and photos/pictures to point to so that the listener can understand the message). Other useful graphics include maps or photographs, menus and newspapers (to point to pictures or written words). High technology aids include software applications on phones, iPads, tablets or laptop computers and electronic communication aids.

Many people with aphasia find it difficult to become independent and effective users of AAC, and you need to consider and match any AAC to a client's language and cognitive profiles, and to present it as something to use alongside other Total Communication strategies. Spoken and written language difficulties, particularly significant comprehension difficulties, make learning and using any AAC challenging. High tech AAC devices often require a good level of cognition and fine motor skills to operate successfully. Any AAC needs to be **at the appropriate level and personalised**: communication boards may not be used because they are too complex, and the vocabulary does not meet clients' needs. An individual's vocabulary is usually best presented in a simple grid display with **clear instructions** for both the person with aphasia and their communication partners as to how to use and update the board or app. It is also essential to have **enough practice** of the AAC (provide simulated practice in therapy sessions and plan real life practice) so that its use becomes an accepted way of communicating. Assessment: it is unclear which people with aphasia should have specialised AAC assessment, so find specialist AAC services for assessment where possible.[3] Some services require people to be able to use a multi-page vocabulary and choose a single symbol/word/phrase or combine them to form a sentence.

PROMOTING APHASIC COMMUNICATIVE EFFECTIVENESS (PACE)

Promoting Aphasic Communicative Effectiveness (PACE) (Davis 2005) is an interactive therapy in which therapy tasks involve the person with aphasia communicating information unknown to the listener, both people give and receive information and any means of getting the message across can be chosen. In this way, the tasks aim to be more like a real life situation, where we don't know what someone wants to say or ask for. It puts the person with aphasia in a position where they need to take responsibility for getting their message across somehow and encourages them to use the strategies available. It puts the listener in the position where they have to listen and watch and focus on the information they are getting and what the message might be. It can involve language games, such as Go Fish which structure the interaction, and using pictures of objects and actions.

82 TOTAL COMMUNICATION

Total Communication provides an opportunity for someone with aphasia to practise communicating using different modalities (speech, writing, gesture, drawing, facial expressions, vocalisations or pointing to pictures or written words) as strategies. It also works to build a process whereby two people work together to piece together partial or incomplete information. For the communication partner to learn how to work out what an incomplete gesture or written word might be, putting that information together with part of a spoken word or facial expression needs practice and support from the SLT. It is helpful for communication partners to learn certain key skills. It is essential for both the person with aphasia and the conversation partner to establish that they will share the responsibility for the success of the conversation and then take on their part. The conversation partner needs to understand that communication may not only involve speech, that it may be incomplete, that it may contain errors and sometimes may be very difficult to understand. They need to learn to listen, to build on partial information, using whatever is offered as a clue to the intended message. This may be linking part of a spoken word with a small gesture. They need to learn to ask for repetition, to check the information given ("Are you saying ...?"), to write down options to clarify the message, to know and use helpful cues. Other essential skills are to know how to repair a conversation when it breaks down, and when to leave the attempt and try later.

Do not assume that every partner or family member will be willing and/or able to learn and use these skills. There may be relationship, personality or cognitive issues that inhibit the use of strategies in conversation. The person with aphasia may also have cognitive deficits (e.g. with working memory, attention, executive functioning) leading to difficulties remembering strategies, moving flexibly between them, combining them and working collaboratively with a communication partner. You may need to model their use repeatedly and provide situations in group therapy where Total Communication is used, observed and practised. Sometimes, a partner may develop skills working with an unfamiliar person with aphasia more easily and may benefit from written reminders and videos to consolidate the information about their role.

MULTI-MODALITY APHASIA THERAPY (M-MAT)

Multi-modality Aphasia Therapy (Rose & Attard 2011) includes treatments using non-verbal modalities (including writing and gesture). These are taught for use in conversation with a total communication approach, and with the aim of improving verbal communication. The theory is that spoken words are facilitated by finding the target word in other modalities. M-MAT uses massed practice (30 hours in two weeks) with encouragement and modifications by the therapist, socially relevant activities and settings (groups). M-MAT builds on cross-modal priming; the use of one modality or strategy helps to promote another modality. It also focuses on encouraging learning, in particular how to support and modify attempts to communicate.

SCRIPT TRAINING

This can be working on the production of a chosen set of words in speech, although some people might add some writing, gestures and drawing and use communication boards in their script. The training utilises phrases rather than single words to create a scripted narrative to use in conversation, perhaps about a holiday, the family or favourite jokes. Like the massed practice done in impairment-based therapy, working on scripts involves working repetitively to learn the words and phrases in clinic and at home and via video-based programmes on computers. The aim is to make the phrases and script more automatic in an everyday conversation, improve communication skills and confidence in everyday situations.

SELF-DISCLOSURE

Some people use scripts to self-disclose their aphasia, which can be an important part of dealing with everyday social interactions. A learned script can be helpful to refer to the aphasia, explain what it is and how the listener can help the interaction progress. Not everyone with aphasia wants or is able to tell people about their aphasia. The social isolation and loss of social activities may mean they are not often in a position where it needs to be explained. Therapy may include supporting your client to consider self-disclosure as a helpful step, and developing a script together to do this makes it a little easier. Clients report that these scripts have helped the interaction by providing enough information for their listeners to react positively and that this increases their confidence to try other conversations.

83 CONVERSATION AND SUPPORT

Conversations are essential for our relationships and well-being. Aphasia therapy that aims to meet a client's everyday communication needs must always address conversation. Conversation therapy focuses on both what the person with aphasia is doing and what their conversation partner is doing in a conversation. Working with someone with aphasia to improve their ability to understand others and to get their message across for everyday conversations usually involves impairment-based assessment and therapy and restoring language functions (at the very least, you need to understand someone's level of auditory and written comprehension to know what type and level of strategy and support will be appropriate), compensatory therapy, learning accessible and functionally useful multi-modal strategies and making the communication environment more conducive to conversations. Using a compensatory approach when working with a client with auditory comprehension difficulties will include building strategies to support their understanding in conversation. Strategies might include reducing distractions, particularly noise in the environment, aiming for more one-to-one conversations where people are face-to-face so that they can benefit from lip-reading and facial expressions and asking people for repetition (using a gesture to indicate this, if not speech). Having a conversation partner who is trained to support someone with aphasia and uses writing, gesture and points at written words or pictures will aid comprehension.

Using strategies in conversation, with someone else supporting any comprehension difficulties and communication attempts, is often referred to as **supported conversation** (Kagan et al. 2001). The principles behind supported conversation are: (1) that someone with aphasia is unable to show their underlying knowledge of the world and social skills (their competence) because the language they need to express them is impaired (this suggests that it is important to acknowledge competence (saying, I know that you know, i.e. I know you have something to say, you are a thinking and competent adult)); (2) that it is possible to help someone reveal their competence, to enable them to understand the conversation and to get their message across using whatever works for them in that situation. Often it is a combination of speech, writing, gesture, pointing, using maps, a newspaper, drawing and communication aids. Rather than the request-response-evaluation sequence that is appropriate for some therapy, supported conversation tries to emulate a 'natural' conversation, with a back-and-forth where both people may initiate or change the direction. While you may need to set up the topic or context in which the conversation is happening, try to put the client in a position where they have the opportunity to control where the conversation goes. A shared activity, such as discussing a national or seasonal event can work in individual or group sessions. The conversation partner (who may be the therapist, family member or volunteer) facilitates and ensures comprehension by using the same strategies (mainly speech and writing), allowing time for language processing and responses.

An important consideration or challenge to **Total Communication** therapy is that when alternative ways of communicating are encouraged, and speech is not worked on, the neural networks responsible for speech production are not used and the subsequent lack of activation weakens the networks further. This **learned non-use** of speech can result when compensatory strategies (e.g. drawing or gesture) are used rather than attempting to use speech to communicate. The hypothesis is that different neural recovery mechanisms are used for speech production and compensatory strategies. In terms of improvements in a client's word retrieval, their functional communication and quality of life, both M-MAT (using Total Communication strategies) and CIAT (which constrains strategies and focuses on speech production) have been shown to be effective (Rose et al. 2022). M-MAT showed more improvement in quality of life and CIAT-plus more improvement in word retrieval.

84 BARRIERS AND RAMPS

Aphasia is more than a language or communication impairment; it is a life-changing event (Duchan & Byng 2004) that brings with it changes in someone's ability to participate in their life. So, therapy also needs to focus on managing long-term communication difficulties and living with the impacts of aphasia, which can result in a loss of autonomy, income, fewer social activities, even social isolation and identity loss (see Chapter 10). This therapy input focuses on the communication environment of someone with aphasia. It looks at how this environment can either prevent or enable them to communicate more easily. Whatever degree of aphasia someone has, it becomes a disability for them if when they try to communicate, their attempts are not met with the support that could enable them to get their message across. In the language of mobility, just as someone in a wheelchair can access a building if there is a ramp, successfully understanding language and getting a message across can depend on whether there are communication 'ramps' or, alternatively, 'barriers' around someone with aphasia.

Barriers prevent someone with aphasia from participating in life. There is little understanding of aphasia in the wider world, there is even a stigma attached to it. Assumptions about lack of speech or disordered speech include judging someone as unintelligent, being mentally unwell or an incompetent adult. The purpose of therapy which adapts the environment of someone with aphasia is to enable them to show their competence and get their message across. Communication may remain an effortful process and need the support of the person listening to them; there may be little spontaneous speech and communicating will involve the use of compensatory strategies, but with someone willing and able to spend the time and learn how to communicate in a different way, someone with aphasia is usually able to get their message across (Kagan 1998).

Part of changing someone's communication environment is training the people around them to become **communication partners**. Communication involves at least two people, so therapy should always include working with both the client and people around them to maximise the success of communication in everyday life. As well as education about aphasia, you can provide **conversation partner training** so that their spouse, family, carers, medical staff and friends are able to support conversation by using remaining speech and compensatory strategies in conversation to enable the person with aphasia to get a message across. While education about aphasia is needed to understand the problems that face successful conversations, supported conversation is about finding solutions to the lack of speech to enable better everyday communication (Wilkinson & Wielaert 2012).

Conversation partners learn about the communication strengths and weaknesses of the client, and about how different strategies can compensate for impaired language skills. It may seem obvious to you but people usually need to see the use of different modalities (including gesture, pointing to written words or pictures or diaries, writing instead of using speech) and use or respond themselves to understand their use. You need to learn to support conversations and model the key elements: acknowledge the intelligence and competence of your client in the way you speak to them and conduct the conversation, actively engage and motivate them in activities and tasks.

For example, it is important that both people in a conversation use gestures and make them a regular part of communication. The conversation partner helps by interpreting and clarifying the gesture, learning how to ask structured questions. Repeated practice is needed for conversation partners to learn about how communication works and new ways to have conversations. You will need to model a conversation that uses strategies to make sure that your client understands what is being communicated to them; model using spoken and written language and other modalities such as pictures or gestures. Provide the means for your client to get their message across, with paper and pen or pictures available. Model using these and allow time, accept silence and partial answers and build on these to get to the intended meaning by checking, clarifying and working together.

This working together can provide a useful balance in the relationship. Now it is not only the client with aphasia who must learn new communication skills, and perhaps find it difficult.

Now both the person with aphasia and their conversation partner have clear tasks to carry out in a conversation. It can be helpful to talk about the balance of responsibility in a conversation; that it is usually 50-50, that aphasia can make it nearly all the responsibility of the conversation partner, but with supported conversation and use of multimodal strategies, the aim is to move towards 50-50. Conversation partners can have their own issues with learning new skills which will need addressing. Some think less flexibly about communication, or about taking on new skills. For most, this is a difficult reminder of the impact of the aphasia on communication and on their relationship. You will need to think about what psychosocial support people would benefit from (see Point 97).

One social model, the Life Participation Approach to Aphasia (**LPAA**) (Chapey et al. 2008) aims to improve life participation, targeting someone with aphasia's long-term needs. It encourages us to focus on functional goals for therapy that improve participation in everyday life and outcomes that measure quality of life. It reminds us that therapy services should be available, whatever the level of impairment, at all stages of someone's life with aphasia. One therapy model using the principles of LPAA is an intensive therapy intervention for people with aphasia after a stroke. **Intensive Comprehensive Aphasia Programs (ICAPs)** involve a minimum of three hours daily therapy over a minimum of two weeks. The therapy includes impairment-based treatments and compensatory therapy, in one-to-one or group formats for the client and partners, communication partner training and education aiming to improve participation in daily activities.

When we focus on how someone is functioning in social situations, we look for whether they use the new communication skills or strategies beyond the clinic situation. This generalisation can be helped by working with their partners and in groups. We can promote **peer befriending**, involving aphasia clients who have experience of living with aphasia and found improvements and ways of managing their communication difficulties. They share experiences and ideas and offer social and emotional support, with empathy. Choosing the right clients to do this needs to be done carefully, with clear expectations and boundaries. **Aphasia group treatment** focuses on building conversation skills and confidence in a group with other people with aphasia. Each person will have their own communication goals (e.g. using writing as a strategy in conversation, asking for repetition of auditory information). The aim is to experience some success communicating with others without aiming for complete accuracy. While you will need to prepare carefully for group sessions and offer a framework that can bolster the flow of the session, the aim is for conversations to evolve as naturally as possible and give practice in managing the ebb and flow/to-and-fro of conversation that can build skills for everyday participation in conversations.

85 DELIVERY OPTIONS

The core of aphasia therapy you will do is direct treatment of the language difficulties (impairment-based and compensatory treatments) via one-to-one sessions, usually face-to-face but also via telehealth (online sessions on the computer or on the telephone using FaceTime). Wherever possible, try and provide your clients with group therapy.

GROUP THERAPY

Group therapy can provide a way of delivering more aphasia therapy when there are constraints on the provision of one-to-one sessions. How long the sessions are and how many you may give will vary. Some models are intensive and short term: CIAT (see above) delivery is 3 hours a day, for 5 days a week, across two weeks (30 hours); an alternative of that model is over 10 weeks. Other groups may involve 1-hour sessions twice a week for 10 weeks (20 hours). You may be able to offer once a week for 1.5 hours for 6 weeks. Whatever is possible in terms of time, make the most of the opportunities that groups offer to your clients. You will need time to plan and prepare the groups, more than you might think. A pro-forma sheet for each client with headings as to what their goals are and specific language and strategy work they are doing is useful; you need to keep careful notes and monitor any progress or changes. Who might you have in a group? In terms of numbers, a group could just be two people, the largest group is usually 6–8. A group of two people (a dyad) involves a different kind of conversation, with more opportunities to speak but fewer opportunities to practise switching attention in conversation and less ebb and flow. The facilitator (SLT or trained volunteer) would take a more active role. It is important to think about what sort of group you are setting up, how it will meet the goals of each individual client, how well matched the clients need to be (in terms of their language skills and difficulties and goals) to be able to work together in the group. If you are aiming for conversations, will it work to have people who have no speech alongside others who are more fluent – what will you need to prepare and do to support everyone in the group to get their message across? Groups where the participants are similar in language profile and in what they are working to improve tend to go more smoothly. You need to consider the personalities of the clients and how well they will get on together, or how you will manage any mismatch of behaviour and expectations. This assumes that you know the group members in advance, which is preferable. With several facilitators or volunteers and options for spaces/rooms, you are better placed to accommodate the different needs of everyone in the group. Aphasia groups may **involve family**, offering peer support from other people living with someone with aphasia and opportunities to share their experiences of aphasia and what has helped manage the changed conversations. It is also an opportunity to provide information about aphasia, about what conversation involves, about ways of improving communication and their important role. There can be more formal training in supported communication and opportunities to practise this both with their partner and other people in the group, with guidance and feedback from the SLT.

The benefits of aphasia groups can be to someone's communication, participation, psychosocial well-being and understanding about aphasia. Group therapy provides the opportunity to use residual speech and non-verbal **communication** strategies in settings where the demands of conversation are nearer to everyday life. Depending on the set-up and number of clinicians available, an aphasia group can provide clients with both individual and group therapy. Each participant in the group can have conversational goals, with language targets (e.g. spoken word production, sentence production, asking questions or understanding questions), strategy-use targets (e.g. using writing, gestures, drawing key words and combining strategies), conversational targets (e.g. initiating conversations, repairing errors or keeping on track). Aphasia groups working on conversation can improve language performance (Hoover et al. 2014) and the use of Total Communication strategies. Group conversations can be more free-flowing than one-to-one interactions and clients can practise the skills needed to participate in conversations, such as initiating, joining in, working out what to contribute and how to do so. An LPAA approach encourages this focus on everyday conversations, increasing successful **participation** in conversations and confidence in communicating. My clients with aphasia often say that one of the biggest aspects of communication that they miss is everyday conversations. Conversation has the potential to connect people; social interaction includes sharing concerns, jokes, listening, telling one's story and offering support and encouragement to others. Group therapy can encourage wider social participation by increasing someone's confidence in their ability to communicate. Conversations with people beyond the family can encourage more independence and connections with the wider world. Encourage people to use the skills developed in aphasia groups to return to groups they belonged to before the aphasia, including looking at the language demands of that group and how to meet and manage those. Being able to regain previous interests and hobbies is important for well-being. Once they have been discharged from hospital, many people with aphasia do not get an opportunity to meet or spend significant time with other people with aphasia. Aphasia groups can help address both the psychological and social needs of your clients. Adapting to the 'new normal' of living with aphasia and the changes this brings in someone's working, social and person life have a significant impact on personal identity. In a group, there is the potential for conversations that are personal, and people often share experiences and emotions. The opportunity to communicate with people who understand the changes and challenges of conversation when you have aphasia provides a community of peers who can support each other. People find that it can be useful to develop a sense of self with aphasia alongside other people who are doing the same. Some people become role models that encourage others (Shadden 2007). **Education** about aphasia and about how to communicate differently/learn new skills can be done in an aphasia-friendly environment; information can be given in an accessible way using supported conversation and adapting spoken and written information to make it accessible (using fewer words, key words or drawings to aid comprehension).

Another important way that therapy is delivered is by the **home practice** you provide. Part of someone's therapy plan must be to make sure that home practice is established, relevant to your client's individual's language profile, therapy goals and personal life. Writing skills can be practised in daily journals, perhaps initially copying words or recording daily life. They can be a set of words for spoken practice, or for script practice, and a record of progress for people to look at. Encourage your clients to think of the practice as work, for some people it is helpful to talk about rehabilitation as their 'new job'. Start with some less challenging work and move on to more difficult tasks. Therapy tasks may involve using therapy apps, paper and pen tasks, self-administered or with help from a trained volunteer, family member or friend. Spend time making sure that the tasks are understood by everyone involved. Suggest scheduling a time or times for the work to be done, to establish a habit, tailoring the tasks into 20- or 30-minute chunks. Some people benefit from having a chart to record or tick off the tasks completed.

86 APHASIA SOFTWARE, COMPUTER THERAPY PROGRAMS, APPS FOR THERAPY

Meeting the challenge of providing therapy with mass practice is helped enormously by computer therapies which can provide hundreds of hours of repetitive practice of therapy tasks. Clients don't have to travel to appointments, can choose when to do their practice, either alone or with help from family/friend/volunteer, and/or with your remote supervision of therapy exercises carried out. Some people need help to access and use the software. Most clients benefit from SLT input during computer therapy programmes, and you need access to the data showing how they are managing the exercises, so you can adapt and revise the therapy programme.

Barriers to using computer therapies include the 'digital divide'; some people have less access to computers due to age, income or education and lack computer literacy. In 2023, only 8 per cent of the adult UK population were non-internet users. However, it is worth noting that 19 per cent of disabled adults were not recent internet users (Ofcom 2023). You many need to help your client connect with local community organisations (e.g. libraries or charities) who provide access and digital skills support. As well as a lack of the necessary support to access computers or apps, where there are cognitive issues, these may be more of a barrier to using technology than the severity of the aphasia. A hemiplegia (paralysis affecting one side of the body) or hemianopia (a visual field deficit with a loss of vision for stimuli in part of the visual field) can also present difficulties navigating screens. There is also the cost and availability of the computer/tablet/ i-Pad and the apps. It can be helpful to start with a simple speech to text software available on phones.

People who have writing difficulties find this useful as they can speak their texts into the phone. Another simple option is a scanning pen, which converts text to speech and reads the text aloud and is helpful for people with reading difficulties.

There are computer-based treatment programmes such as the Sentence Production Treatment (Hickin, Cruice & Dipper 2022) which is delivered via both face-to-face therapy with an SLT and independent work by the client. It involves treatment of verbs, sentences and generalisation. An example of a therapy using digital technology is EVA Park (Marshall et al. 2016). This is a multi-user, online virtual island. It contains several virtual locations, such as houses and shops. The people with aphasia are represented by avatars and use speech to communicate with each other and with therapists. It provides an opportunity to practise speech in social situations, and to build connections with other people with aphasia. ORLA (Cherney 2010) uses either an avatar therapist or live SLT to deliver a treatment for reading. It involves 24 sessions of treatment 1–3 times per week. Aphasia Scripts (Lee , Kaye & Cherney 2009) is a programme designed for script practice and uses a personal animated therapist (PAT).

There are a large number of aphasia therapy apps offering exercises to work on such areas as word retrieval, understanding single words and sentences, reading, writing and sentence production. Look for apps that are evidence-based, easy to use and accessible to people regardless of the severity of their aphasia. Consider the cost (some are free, some are provided by charities). Try to find ones that have clear, short presentations of the therapy tasks and how to select words and levels. Some apps change the difficulty of tasks automatically as appropriate. Look for those with a large number of exercises and lexical items, where there are different cueing possibilities and you can select the items to be practised and change the exercises, increasing or decreasing the level as appropriate. Some apps change the difficulty of tasks automatically. It is useful for your client to have immediate feedback when they work on an exercise. Can you upload someone's photos to make the exercises personal? Are the images used clear, with photos rather than line drawings and with few visual distractions in any pictures? Can the font size be increased? Is the voice used on the app a natural voice? Can you adjust the rate of speech delivery? Are there exercises beyond single word level, with therapy for sentence and or discourse level? See links in Appendix 5, particularly the Aphasia Software Finder, a very useful source of information on the therapy apps and software available. It is accessible for people with aphasia, so you can recommend it to clients as well as using it yourself.

87 TELEHEALTH

Telehealth is also referred to as telerehabilitation or online therapy, this method of delivery became more widely used during the Covid-19 pandemic when ways of providing therapy other than face-to-face were needed. Now, it is more acceptable as an option to provide therapy that is long-distance and more accessible for people with mobility or fatigue issues who find the journey to clinic difficult and tiring. Your professional regulator, workplace or insurance provider will have regulations and policies regarding telehealth practice to ensure that it respects confidentiality, manages risk and maintains security, follows current legislation and promotes and safeguards the interests of clients and carers.

If we need to monitor our client's general well-being, progress and engagement in an existing rehabilitation programme, then a phone call or text messaging (SMS) is one option, depending on the client's communication abilities. It can also be used to support engagement and provide simple education. Many people with aphasia use FaceTime or WhatsApp with family and friends and these provide the lip-reading and visual cues that help communication. Videoconferencing can be used to deliver a therapy programme, for example, to observe function, perform assessments remotely or demonstrate and modify exercises. Many platforms have whiteboard, screen sharing and file sharing functions, which can be useful features. Web-based links, video and PDFs of educational and rehabilitation activities can be shared via email or text. It is also possible to quickly develop and share video resources to groups and individual clients.

There can be issues which you should make your client aware of; increased exposure to privacy and digital security risks, technical problems causing delays, reduced visual and sound quality for observations and modelling. Some clients do not like working in this way, reporting that it is not the same as a face-to-face session. You may find that some clients and/or some treatments do not work well online. Many people need help from a family member at the start and end of a session to help with technical set up and during the session to use multiple modalities, e.g. gesture (thumbs up, pointing to written words, objects or pictures), writing, with either pen and paper held up to the camera, a whiteboard or screen-sharing. You can also use a visualiser (e.g. Hue camera)[4] to show words/drawing for assessment and therapy.

People need time to feel comfortable online and familiar with the various controls at the start of the session. It is helpful to factor in time for breaks (turn off the camera for ten minutes to get a cup of tea or use the loo). Spending time ensuring your client has the necessary skills to use online platforms is part of therapy; these are skills that can be used outside therapy sessions to connect with other people for conversations online. Your client may find it helpful to remove the self-view function during sessions; seeing yourself when speaking is not part of normal conversation and can be distracting or even disconcerting.

ON DELIVERY

Involve everyone you can to promote and carry out therapy practice and find out which therapy tasks a client can do on their own and which they need help with from someone at home. This can involve training other people (family members, friends, volunteers, SLT assistants) to understand the aphasia and the treatment plan, and to carry out therapy tasks. We need to check how the therapy practice is being carried out, monitor and measure and adjust tasks to make them more accessible and/or challenging.

88 THERAPY GAINS: GENERALISATION

When we ask whether it works or not, we are thinking of gains made in treatment that to go beyond the treatment session to improve everyday communication. Generalisation is dependent on therapy being successful. We look for whether a client can use the treated language or strategy outside the therapy session and whether there is any improvement beyond what has been targeted in treatment. This 'generalisation' is a key aim of therapy. There is more likely to be generalisation when you target an underlying language process as well as a set of words. So, therapy to improve spoken word production working on phonological and/or semantic skills may improve word retrieval for words you have not targeted in therapy (Madden, Torrence & Kendall 2020). There may be less generalisation of trained words or strategies in everyday conversations (Greenwood et al. 2010). Think about how single words can be used in discourse, in conversations, when you design therapy. Look at whether someone's language and cognitive skills are adequate to meet the demands of the controlled environment of the therapy session, and whether the different challenges of everyday conversations need to be considered and be a target of therapy. Perhaps there are attention, auditory memory and/or comprehension difficulties that need working on for them to be able to participate in conversations. Increase the situations in which someone uses the language worked on from one-to-one conversations to group settings. Many group therapy structures provide this format, with time for individuals to work on their targets and opportunities for them to practise in group conversations. Working on creating scripts may be useful for encouraging the use of the target words beyond single word level; building phrases from targeted words and practising these as scripts can improve their use in conversation.

MAINTAINING THERAPY GAINS

We aim for our clients to maintain the improvements they make from language therapy, which may be seen both in language processing scores and in someone's ability to participate in conversation, e.g. ICAP (Leff et al. 2021) where such gains continued in the three months after the therapy programme. How do we help people maintain the progress they make in their communication beyond therapy? Include the issue of maintenance in your therapy provision; part of the education around aphasia and rehabilitation should include understanding the importance of maintaining improvements made during therapy and how to do so. The support people may need includes access to services, which might entail further therapy input, regular reviews and more treatment, support from aphasia charities and groups (see links in Appendix 5), support from family and friends, including supported conversation. Continued, regular home practice of targeted therapy will also be necessary, as will opportunities to communicate successfully despite the aphasia, particularly in personally meaningful conversations. Making sure these conversations are a regular part of someone's everyday life may be key to maintenance of gains (Menahemi-Falkove et al. 2024).

COMBINING THERAPIES

> After his stroke (a large left MCA territory infarct) Ben had very little speech – just one or two recurring utterances. He could not produce spoken words in response to conversational questions, pictures, repetition or as automatic (serial) speech. He had some auditory and reading comprehension difficulties. He did not use gesture or writing spontaneously. Assessment showed better skills with written language than spoken, with better reading comprehension and more writing than speech. He

had a communication chart on his iPad which he did not use. While he and his wife wanted to work on restoring speech from the beginning of therapy, it was explained to them that this work would be slow and that it would be useful to work both on his speech and on other ways of getting his message across. Therapy sessions initially involved working on writing, using an impairment-based approach and included setting up daily practice using apps to build his ability to write words in response to pictures and to the spoken word (given the letters) and written word to picture matching tasks. Therapy also involved working on gesture and on the use of the communication chart. A combination of writing, drawing, gesture and the communication chart was worked on with a compensatory approach (Total Communication). Therapy included PACE activities. Speech was encouraged along with these tasks but it took several months before he had any control over speech production, helped by writing. Therapy then continued with both the compensatory approach, to help with conversation and to promote speech, and an impairment approach using semantic and phonological therapy to target underlying language processes.

Following his stroke, Bob had some speech, but it was effortful and slow with frequent pauses, word errors and incomplete sentences. He struggled to initiate conversations and to take part in them. He was becoming more and more unwilling to try and communicate. He could write a little more easily than he could speak but was not comfortable with using writing when it was suggested. He didn't always follow what his wife Sheila said to him and would get the wrong things out of the drawer, for example. All this information came from the first appointment, from initial observations, informal assessment and reports from Bob and his wife. Further assessment showed more about the word retrieval difficulties and the auditory comprehension deficits. Bob's goals were to get back into conversations with more speech, to try writing, to understand Sheila better day-to-day. The initial therapy included impairment-based treatment for his word retrieval, including verb comprehension and production, phonological and semantic therapy with a set of 150 words relevant to Bob's everyday life. A compensatory approach encouraged the use of writing in tasks and as a strategy in conversations in clinic with carry-over into conversations at home. It also worked on narrative therapy, where Bob and Sheila prepared short phrases and paragraphs of things Bob might want to say in the course of an average day, including 'Hello, Mike!' and 'We went to Bridlington on Saturday' to encourage participation in conversations. Therapy to address Bob's environment involved ensuring that Sheila was an active participant in the sessions, that she learned about aphasia and had training in supported conversation techniques with Bob. She was able to pass on this information and training to family and friends who had conversations with him. As Bob's ability to use speech and writing to communicate in everyday conversations developed, he wanted to improve his speech production and further assessment revealed more about his anomia and targeted further impairment-based therapy. Bob moved cities but wrote frequent postcards from his travels and sent photos of him smiling, sitting with friends.

Mrs. B missed playing golf. She was now reluctant to play because she was concerned that she would not be able to talk to her friends easily as they went round the course; in particular that she would have word retrieval difficulties for the everyday 'golfing' words she would need. She was embarrassed and anxious and avoiding golf altogether. Therapy involved education about aphasia and her language difficulties. An impairment-based therapy programme included agreeing the words and phrases she might need, designing semantic and phonological therapy tasks to improve word retrieval for those words (including picture-matching, picture-written word matching, repetition of target words and narrative writing). Consequence/compensatory therapy involved building strategies for managing word retrieval difficulties in conversation. Mrs. B could use written forms of the words practised and we created a card that she took with her on the golf course. She put it with her golf card. Discussions about this revealed her difficulties with numbers (when writing her score on the card); this was contributing to her feelings of discomfort. Therapy then included assessment and impairment-based therapy for numbers and arithmetic. Therapy for the environment looked at the need for the people around her to support and enable her to communicate more easily; including involving some friends with education about aphasia, her difficulties and concerns and how they could help her. One friend was very keen to help and came to some SLT sessions to learn more about aphasia and supported conversation techniques and how to support Mrs. B in conversation.

NOTES

1 https://www.nice.org.uk/guidance/qs2/chapter/Quality-statement-2-Intensity-of-stroke-rehabilitation.
2 https://nadiiatherapy.com
3 https://assistivetechnology.org.uk
4 https://huehd.com/apps

REFERENCES

Ball, A. L., de Riesthal, M., Breeding, V. E., & Mendoza, D. E. (2011). Modified ACT and CART in severe aphasia. *Aphasiology,* 25(6–7): 836–848.

Basso, A., Capitani, E., Vignolo, L. A. (1979). Influence of rehabilitation on language skills in aphasic patients: a controlled study. *Archives of Neurology,* 36(4): 190–196.

Bhogal, S., Teasell, R., Speechley, M., & Albert, M. L. (2003). Intensity of aphasia therapy, impact on recovery. *Stroke,* 34(4): 987–993.

Boyle, M. (2010). Semantic feature analysis treatment for aphasic word retrieval impairments: what's in a name? *Topics in Stroke Rehabilitation,* 17(6): 411–422. https://doi.org/10.1310/tsr1706-411

Brady, M. C., Kelly, H., Godwin, J., Enderby, P., & Campbell, P. (2016, 1 June). Speech and language therapy for aphasia following stroke (Review). *Cochrane Database of Systematic Reviews.* https://doi.org/10.1002/14651858

Chapey, R., Duchan, J. F., Elman, R. J., Garcia, L. J., Kagan, A., Lyon, J. G., & Simmons-Mackie, N. (2008). Life-participation approach to aphasia: a statement of values for the future. In R. Chapey (Ed.), *Language Intervention Strategies in Aphasia and Related Neurogenic Communication Disorders* (pp. 279–289). Lippincott Williams & Wilkins.

Cherney, L. R. (2010) Oral Reading for Language in Aphasia (ORLA): evaluating the efficacy of computer-delivered therapy in chronic nonfluent aphasia. *Topics in Stroke Rehabilitation,* 17(6): 423–431. https://www.sralab.org/aphasiasoftware

Davis, G. A. (2005). PACE revisited. *Aphasiology,* 19(1): 21–38. https://doi.org/10.1080/02687030444000598

Dipper, L., Devane, N., Barnard, R., Botting, N., Boyle, M., Cockayne, L., Hersh, D., Magdalani, C., Marshall, J., Swinburn, K., & Cruice, M. (2024). A feasibility randomised waitlist-controlled trial of a personalised multi-level language treatment for people with aphasia: the remote LUNA study. *PLoS One.* 19(6): e0304385. doi:10.1371/journal.pone.0304385

Duchan, J. F., & Byng, S. (Eds.). (2004) *Challenging Aphasia Therapies: Broadening the Discourse and Extending the Boundaries.* Taylor & Francis.

Edmonds, L. A., Mammino, K., & Ojeda, J. (2014). Effect of verb network strengthening treatment (VNeST) in persons with aphasia: extension and replication of previous findings. *American Journal of Speech-Language Pathology*, 23(2): 312–329. doi: 10.1044/2014_AJSLP-13-0098.

Greenwood, A., Grassly, J., Hickin, J., & Best, W. (2010). Phonological and orthographic cueing therapy: a case of generalised improvement. *Aphasiology*, 24(9): 991–1016. https://doi.org/10.1080/02687030903168220

Heath, C., Conroy, P., Pellegrini, I., & Bruehl, S. (2022). Investigating the neural basis of post-stroke aphasia therapy; a systematic review of neuroscience-based therapy studies. *Aphasiology* (9): 1508–1532. doi: https://doi.org/10.1080/02687038.2022.2101089

Hebb, D. O. (1949). *The Organization of Behaviour; a Neuropsychological Theory*. Wiley.

Herbert, R., Best, W., Hickin, J., Howard, D., & Osborne, F. (2003). Combining lexical and interactional approaches to therapy for word finding deficits in aphasia. *Aphasiology*, 17(12): 1163–1186. doi: 10.1080/02687030344000454

Hickin, J., Cruice, M., & Dipper, L. (2022). A feasibility study of a novel computer-based treatment for sentence production deficits in aphasia, delivered by a combination of clinician-led and self-managed treatment sessions. *Aphasiology*, 37(10): 1623–1645. https://doi.org/10.1080/02687038.2022.2116928

Kagan, A. (1998). Supported conversation for adults with aphasia: methods and resources for training conversation partners. *Aphasiology*, 12(9): 816–830. doi:10.1080/02687039808249575

Kagan, A., Black, S. E., Duchan, F. J., Simmons-Mackie, N., Square, P. (2001).Training volunteers as conversation partners using "Supported Conversation for Adults with Aphasia" (SCA): a controlled trial. *Journal of Speech, Language and Hearing Research*, 44(3): 624–638. doi: 10.1044/1092-4388(2001/051).

Kistner, J., Dipper, L. T., & Marshall, J. (2018). The use and function of gestures in word-finding difficulties in aphasia. *Aphasiology*, 33(11): 1372–1392. https://doi.org/10.1080/02687038.2018.1541343

Lee, J. B., Kaye, R. C., & Cherney, L. R. (2009). Conversational script performance in adults with non-fluent aphasia: treatment intensity and aphasia severity. *Aphasiology*, 23(7–8): 885–897. https://doi.org/10.1080/02687030802669534

Leff, A. P., Nightingale, S., Gooding, B., Rutter, J., Craven, N., Peart, M., Dunstan, A., Sherman, A., Paget, A., Duncan, M., Davidson, J., Kumar, N., Farrington-Douglas, C., Julien, C., & Crinion, J.

T. (2021). Clinical effectiveness of the Queen's Square intensive comprehensive aphasia service for patients with poststroke aphasia. *Stroke*, 52(10): e594-e598. https://doi.org/10.1161/strokeaha.120.033837

Leonard, C., Rochon, E., & Laird, L. (2008). Treating naming impairments in aphasia: findings from a phonological components analysis treatment. *Aphasiology*, 22(9): 923–947. https://doi.org/10.1080/02687030701831474

Lum, C. (2002) *Scientific Thinking in Speech and Language Therapy*. Lawrence Erlbaum Associates.

Madden, E. B., Torrence, J., & Kendall, D. L. (2020). Cross-modal generalization of anomia treatment to reading in aphasia. *Aphasiology*, 35(7): 875–899. https://doi.org/10.1080/02687038.2020.1734529

Marshall, J. (1995). The mapping hypothesis and aphasia therapy. *Aphasiology*, 9(6): 517–539.

Marshall, J., Booth, T., Devane, N., Galliers, J., Greenwood, H., Hilari, K., Talbot, R., Wilson, S., & Woolf, C. (2016). Evaluating the benefits of aphasia intervention delivered in virtual reality: results of a quasi-randomised study. *PLoS ONE*, 11(8): e0160381. https://doi.org/10.1371/journal.pone.0160381

Menahemi-Falkov, M., O'Halloran, R., Hill, A. J., & Rose, M. L. (2024). *"I've got no skills to maintain – to keep that going"*: a qualitative study of people with chronic aphasia and their partners about factors contributing to the maintenance of aphasia therapy gains. *Aphasiology*, 1–24. https://doi.org/10.1080/02687038.2024.2356875

Molino, M., Egan, A., & Kuschmann, A. (2024). The impact of a university-based intensive comprehensive aphasia programme (ICAP) on language, functional communication and quality of life in people with chronic aphasia. *Aphasiology*, 1–20. https://doi.org/10.1080/02687038.2024.2368623

Monnelly, K., Marshall, J., & Cruice, M. (2021). Intensive comprehensive aphasia programmes: a systematic scoping review and analysis using the TIDieR checklist for reporting interventions. *Disability and Rehabilitation*, 44(21): 6471–6496. https://doi.org/10.1080/09638288.2021.1964626

Ofcom. (2023). Adults' Media Use and Attitudes Report. https://www.ofcom.org.uk/siteassets/resources/documents/research-and-data/media-literacy-research/adults/adults-media-use-and-attitudes-2023/adults-media-use-and-attitudes-report-2023.pdf?v=329409

Palmer, R., Hughes, H., & Chater, T. (2017). What do people with aphasia want to be able to say? A content analysis of words identified as personally relevant by people with aphasia. *PLoS One*, 12(3): e0174065. doi: 10.1371/journal.pone.0174065.

Palmer, R., Witts, H., Chater, T. (2018). What speech and language therapy do community dwelling stroke survivors with aphasia receive in the UK? *PLoS ONE*, 13(7): e0200096. https://doi.org/10.1371/journal.pone.0200096

Pulvermüller, F., Neininger, B., Elbert, T., Mohr, B., Rockstroh, B., Koebbel, P., Taub, E. (2001). Constraint-induced therapy of chronic aphasia after stroke. *Stroke*, 32(7): 1621–1626. doi: 10.1161/01.str.32.7.1621

Rose, M. L. (2013). Releasing the constraints on aphasia therapy: the positive impact of gesture and multimodality treatments. *American Journal of Speech-Language Pathology*, 22(2): S227–S239. https://doi.org/10.1044/1058-0360(2012/12-0091

Rose, M., & Attard, M. (2011). *Multi-modality Aphasia Therapy: A Treatment Manual*. La Trobe University, Melbourne, Australia.

Rose, M. L., Pierce, J. E., Scharp, V. L., Off, C. A., Babbitt, E. M., Griffin-Musick, J. R. & Cherney, L. R. (2022). Developments in the application of intensive comprehensive aphasia programs: an international survey of practice. *Disability and Rehabilitation*, 44(20): 5863–5877. doi: 10.1080/09638288.2021.1948621

Rose, M. L., Raymer, A. M., Lanyon, L. E., & Attard, M. C. (2013). A systematic review of gesture treatments for post-stroke aphasia. *Aphasiology*, 27(9):1090–1127. doi:10.1080/02687038.2013.826473

Shadden, B. (2007). Rebuilding identity through stroke support groups: embracing the person with aphasia and significant others. In R. Elman (Ed.), *Group Treatment of Neurogenic Communication Disorders: The Expert Clinician's Approach*, 2nd ed. (pp. 111–126). Plural Publishers.

Simmons-Mackie, N., Worrall, L., Murray, L. L., Enderby, P., Rose, M. L., Paek, E. J., & Klippi, A. on behalf of the Aphasia United Best Practices Working Group and Advisory Committee. (2017). The top ten: best practice recommendations for aphasia. *Aphasiology*, 31(2): 131–151. doi: 10.1080/02687038.2016.1180662 https://doi.org/10.1080/02687038.2016.1180662

Swinburn, K., Porter, G., Howard D. (2023). *The Comprehensive Aphasia Test (CAT*, 2nd ed. Routledge.

Thomas, L., Lander, L., Cox, N., & Romani, C. (2020). Speech and language therapy for aphasia: parameters and outcomes.

Aphasiology, 34(5): 603–642. https://doi.org/10.1080/02687038.2020.1712588

Webster, J., Morris, J., Whitworth, A., & Howard, D. (2009). *Newcastle University Aphasia Therapy Resources.* Newcastle: The University of Newcastle upon Tyne.

Webster, J., & Whitworth, A. (2012). Treating verbs in aphasia: exploring the impact of therapy at the single word and sentence levels. *International Journal of Language and Communication Disorders*, 47(6): 619–636. doi: 10.1111/j.1460-6984.2012.00174.x

Wilkinson, R., & Wielaert, S. (2012). Rehabilitation targeted at everyday communication: can we change the talk of people with aphasia and their significant others within conversation? *Archives of Physical Medicine and Rehabilitation*, 93(1Suppl.): S7076. doi: 10.1016/j.apmr.2011.07.206

Yamaji, C., & Maeshima, S. (2022). Spontaneous recovery and intervention in aphasia. *Aphasia Compendium.* Intech Open. doi: 10.5772/intechopen.100851

FURTHER READING

Allen, L., Mehta, S., McClure, J. A., & Teasell, R. (2012). Therapeutic interventions for aphasia initiated more than six months post stroke: a review of the evidence. *Topics in Stroke Rehabilitation*, 19(6): 523–535. doi: https://doi.org/10.1310/tsr1906-523

Baker, E. (2012). Optimal intervention intensity. *International Journal of Speech-Language Pathology*, 14(5): 401–409. https://doi.org/10.3109/17549507.2012.700323

Ball, A. L., de Riesthal, M., Breeding, V. E., & Mendoza, D. E. (2011). Modified ACT and CART in severe aphasia. *Aphasiology*, 25(6–7): 836–848.

Basso, A. (2003). *Aphasia and Its Therapy.* Oxford University Press.

Basso, A., & Macis, M. (2011). Therapy efficacy in chronic aphasia. Behavioural Neurology, 24(4): 317–325. doi: https://doi.org/10.3233/BEN-2011-0342

Battye, A. (2023). *Navigating AAC.* Routledge.

Baxter, S., Enderby, P., Evans, P., & Judge, S. (2012). Interventions using high-technology communication devices: a state-of-the-art review. *Folia Phoniatrica et Logopaedica*, 64(3): 137–144. doi: 10.1159/000338250

Beeke, S. & Bloch, S. (.). (2023). *Better Conversations with Communication Difficulties: A Practical Guide for Clinicians.* J&R Press.

Beeson, P., Rising, K., & Volk, J. (2003). Writing treatment for severe aphasia: who benefits? *Journal of Speech, Language and Hearing Research*, 46: 1038–1060.

Bernstein-Ellis, E., & Elman, R. (2007). Aphasia communication group treatment: the aphasia center of California approach. In R. Elman (Ed.), *Group Treatment for Neurogenic Communication Disorders: The Expert Clinician's Approach*, 2nd ed. Plural Publishing.

Bilda, K. (2010). Video-based conversational script training for aphasia: a therapy study. *Aphasiology*, 25(2): 191–201. https://doi.org/10.1080/02687031003798254

Boyle, M. (2011). Discourse treatment for word retrieval impairment in aphasia: the story so

Brogan, E., Ciccone, N., & Godecke, E. (2020). An exploration of aphasia therapy dosage in the first six months of stroke recovery. *Neuropsychological Rehabilitation*, 31(8): 1254–1288. https://doi.org/10.1080/09602011.2020.1776135

Byng, S., Duchan, J., Pound, C. (2007). *The Aphasia Therapy File*, Volume 2. Psychology Press.

Byng, S., Swinburn, K., Pound, C. (1999). *The Aphasia Therapy File*. Psychology Press.

Carragher, M., Conroy, P., Sage, K., & Wilkinson, R. (2012). Can impairment-focused therapy change the everyday conversations of people with aphasia? A review of the literature and future directions. *Aphasiology*, 26(7): 895–916. doi: 10.1080/02687038.2012.676164

Carragher, M., Sage, K., & Conroy, P. (2015). Outcomes of treatment targeting syntax production in people with Broca's-type aphasia: evidence from psycholinguistic assessment tasks and everyday conversation. *International Journal of Language & Communication Disorders*, 50(3): 322–336. https://doi.org/10.1111/1460-6984.12135

Caute, A., Pring, T., Cocks, N., Cruice, M., Best, W., & Marshall, J. (2013). Enhancing communication through gesture and naming therapy. *Journal of Speech, Language and Hearing Research*, 56: 337–351. https://doi.org/10.1044/1092-4388(2012/11-0232

Cherney, L. R., & van Vuuren, S. (2012). Telerehabilitation, virtual therapists, and acquired neurologic speech and language disorders. *Seminars in Speech and Language*, 33(3g): 243–257. doi: 10.1055/s-0032-1320044

Coppens, P., & Patterson, J. (2018). *Aphasia Rehabilitation Clinical Challenges*. Jones and Bartlett. (See Chapter 7.)

Cuperus, P., de Kok, D., de Aguiar, V., & Nickels, L. (2022). Understanding user needs for digital aphasia therapy: experiences and preferences of speech and language therapists. *Aphasiology*, 37(7): 1016–1038. https://doi.org/10.1080/02687038.2022.2066622https://evapark.city.ac.uk

Dahlberg, C. A., Cusick, C. P., Hawley, L. A., Newman, J. K., Morey, C. E., Harrison-Felix, C. L., & Whiteneck, G. G. (2007). Treatment efficacy of social communication skills training after traumatic brain injury: a randomized treatment and deferred treatment-controlled trial. *Archives of Physical Medicine and Rehabilitation*, 88(12): 1561–1573.

Davies, R. (2023). *Navigating Telehealth for Speech and Language Therapists*. Routledge.

de Kleine, N., Rose, M. L., Weinborn, M., Knox, R., & Fay, N. (2023). Does gesture improve the communication success of people with aphasia?: A systematic review. *Aphasiology*, 38(3): 462–486. https://doi.org/10.1080/02687038.2023.2207781

Duchan, J. F., & Byng, S. (Eds.). (2004) *Challenging Aphasia Therapies: Broadening the Discourse and Extending the Boundaries*. Taylor & Francis.

Edmonds, L. A., Mammino, K., & Ojeda, J. (2014). Effect of verb network strengthening treatment (VNeST) in persons with aphasia: extension and replication of previous findings. *American Journal of Speech-Language Pathology*, 23(2): 312–329. doi: 10.1044/2014_AJSLP-13-0098.

Elman, R. J. (Ed.). (2007) *Group Treatment of Neurogenic Communication Disorders: The Expert Clinician's Approach*, 2nd ed. Plural.

Elman, R. J., & Bernstein-Ellis, E. (1999). The efficacy of group communication treatment in adults with chronic aphasia. *Journal of Speech, Language, and Hearing Research*, 42(2): 411–419. https://doi.org/10.1044/jslhr.4202.411

Francis, D. R., Riddoch, M. J., & Humphreys, G. W. (2001). Cognitive rehabilitation of word meaning deafness. *Aphasiology*, 15(8): 749–766. https://doi.org/10.1080/02687040143000177

Franklin, S., Buerk, F., & Howard, D. (2002). Generalised improvement in speech production for a subject with reproduction conduction aphasia. *Aphasiology*, 16(10–11): 1087–1114.

Galletta, E. E., Barrett, A. M. (2014). Impairment and functional interventions for aphasia: having it all. *Current Physical Medical Rehabilitation Reports*, 2(2): 114–120. doi: 10.1007/s40141-014-0050-5.

Hart, T., Dijkers, M. P., Whyte, J., Turkstra, L. S., Zanca, J. M., Packel, A., Van Stan, J. H., Ferraro, M., Chen, C. (2019). A theory-driven system for the specification of rehabilitation treatments. *Archives of Physical Medicine and Rehabilitation*, 100(1): 172–180. doi: 10.1016/j.apmr.2018.09.109. :

Hogrefe, K., Ziegler, W., Weidinger, N., & Goldenberg, G. (2012). Non-verbal communication in severe aphasia: influence of aphasia, apraxia, or semantic processing? *Cortex*, 48(8): 952–962. doi: 10.1016/j.cortex.2011.02.022

Holland, A. D., Fromm, D., Forbes, M., & MacWhinney, B. (2016). Long-term recovery in stroke companied by aphasia: a reconsideration. *Aphasiology*, 31(2): 152–165 doi: 10.1080/02687038.2016.1184221

Hoover, E. L., Caplan, D., Waters, G., & Budson, A. (2014). Effects of impairment-based individual and socially oriented group therapies on verb production in aphasia. *Aphasiology*, 29(7): 781–798. https://doi.org/10.1080/02687038.2014.989953

Hoover, E. L., Caplan, D., Waters, G., & Budson, A. (2015) Effects of impairment-based individual and socially oriented group therapies on verb production in aphasia. *Aphasiology*, 29(7): 781–798. doi: 10.1080/02687038.2014.989953

Howard, D., & Hatfield, F. (1987). *Aphasia Therapy: Historical and Contemporary Issues*. Lawrence Erlbaum Associates Ltd.

Husak, R. S., Wallace, S. E., Marshall, R. C., & Visch-Brink, E. V. (2021). A systematic review of aphasia therapy provided in the early period of post-stroke recovery. *Aphasiology*, 37(1): 143–176. doi: 10.1080/02687038.2021.1987381

Kagan A. (2011). A-FROM in action at the Aphasia Institute. *Seminars in Speech and Language*, 32(3): 216–228. doi: 10.1055/s-0031-1286176

Kagan, A.,& Gailey, G. F. (1993). Functional is not enough: training conversation partners for aphasic adults. In A. L. Holland and M. M. Forbes (Eds.), *Aphasia Treatment: World Perspectives* (pp.199–225). Springer Publishing Group, Inc.

Kaye, R. C., Cherney, L. R. (2016). Script templates: a practical approach to script training in aphasia. *Topics in Language Disorders*, ;36(2): 136–153. doi: 10.1097/TLD.0000000000000086.

Kelly, H. & Armstrong, L. (2009). New word learning in people with aphasia. *Aphasiology*, 23(12): 1398–1417. https://doi.org/10.1080/02687030802289200

Kelly, H., Kennedy, F., Britton, H., McGuire, G., & Law, J. (2016). Narrowing the "digital divide"—facilitating access to computer technology to enhance the lives of those with aphasia: a feasibility study. *Aphasiology*, 30(2–3): 133–163. doi: 10.1080/02687038.2015.1077926

Kiran, S., Thompson, C. K., & Hashimoto, N. (2001). Training grapheme to phoneme conversion in patients with oral reading and naming deficits: a model-based approach. *Aphasiology*, 15(9): 855–876. https://doi.org/10.1080/02687040143000258

Königs, M., Beurskens, E. A., Snoep, L., Scherder, E. J., & Oosterlaan, J. (2018). Effects of timing and intensity of neurorehabilitation on functional outcome after traumatic brain injury: a systematic review and meta-analysis. *Archives of Physical Medicine and Rehabilitation*, 99(6): 1149–1159.

Kurland, J., Liu, A., & Stokes, P. (2018). Effects of a tablet-based home practice program with telepractice on treatment outcomes in chronic aphasia. *Journal of Speech, Language, and Hearing Research*, 61(5): 1140–1156. doi:10.1044/2018_JSLHR-L-17-0277

Laine, M., & Martin, N. (2024). *Anomia: Theoretical and Clinical Aspects*, 2nd ed. Routledge.

Lambon, R. M. A., Snell, C., Fillingham, J. K., Conroy, P., & Sage, K. (2010). Predicting the outcome of anomia therapy for people with aphasia post CVA: both language and cognitive status are key predictors. *Neuropsychological Rehabilitation*, 20(2): 289–305.

Lanyon, L., & Rose, M. L. (2009). Do the hands have it? the facilitation effects of arm and hand gesture on word retrieval in aphasia. *Aphasiology*, 23(7–8): 809–822. doi: 10.1080/02687030802642044

Lanyon, L. E., Rose, M. L., & Worrall, L. (2013). The efficacy of outpatient and community-based aphasia group interventions: a systematic review. *International Journal of Speech-Language Pathology*, 15(4): 359–374. doi: 10.3109/17549507.2012.752865

Lavoie, M., Bier, N., & Macoir, J. (2019). Efficacy of a self-administered treatment using a smart tablet to improve functional vocabulary in post-stroke aphasia: a case-series study. *International Journal of Language & Communication Disorders*, 54: 249–264. https://doi.org/10.1111/1460-6984.12439

Lavoie, M., Macoir, J., & Bier, N. (2017). Effectiveness of technologies in the treatment of post stroke anomia: a systematic review. *Journal of Communication Disorders*, 65: 43–53. https://doi.org/10.1016/j.jcomdis.2017.01.001 PMID: 28171741

Lee, J. B., Kaye, R. C., & Cherney, L. R. (2009). Conversational script performance in adults with non-fluent aphasia: treatment intensity and aphasia severity. *Aphasiology*, 23(7–8): 885–897. https://doi.org/10.1080/02687030802669534

Leonard, C., Rochon, E., & Laird, L. (2008). Treating naming impairments in aphasia: findings from a phonological components analysis treatment. *Aphasiology*, 22(9): 923–947. https://doi.org/10.1080/02687030701831474

Levelt, W. J. M. (1999). Producing spoken language: a blueprint of the speaker. In C. M. Brown & P. Hagoort (Eds.), *The Neurocognition of Language* (pp. 83–122). Oxford University Press.

Maeshima, S., Okamoto, S., Sonoda, S., Osawa, A. (2014). Data analysis of recovery from aphasia with stroke. *Higher Brain Function Research*, 34(3): 298–304.

Marshall, J. (2009). Framing ideas in aphasia: the need for thinking therapy. *International Journal of Language & Communication Disorders*, 44(1): 1–4. https://doi.org/10.1080/13682820802683507

Marshall, J., & Cairns, D. (2005). Therapy for sentence processing problems in aphasia: working on thinking for speaking. *Aphasiology*, 19(10–11): 1009–1020. https://doi.org/10.1080/02687030544000218

Marshall, J., Caute, A., Chadd, K., Cruice, M., Monnelly, K., Wilson, S., & Woolf, C. (2019). Technology-enhanced writing therapy for people with aphasia: results of a quasi-randomized waitlist controlled study. *International Journal of Language & Communication Disorders*, 54(2): 203–220. https://doi.org/10.1111/1460-6984.12391

Martin, N., Thompson, C. K., & Worrall, L. (2008). *Aphasia Rehabilitation: The Impairment and Its Consequences* Plural Publishing Inc.

Miniussi, C., & Giuseppe Vallar (2011) Brain stimulation and behavioural cognitive rehabilitation: a new tool for neurorehabilitation? *Neuropsychological Rehabilitation*, 21(5): 553–559. https://doi.org/10.1080/09602011.2011.622435

Nickels, L. (2002). Therapy for naming disorders: revisiting, revising, and reviewing. *Aphasiology*, 16(10–11): 935–979. https://doi.org/10.1080/02687030244000563

Parr, S., Byng S., Gilpin, S., Ireland, C. (1997). *Talking about Aphasia: Living with Loss of Language after Stroke*. Open University Press.

Pattee, C., Von Berg, S., & Ghezzi, P. (2006). Effects of alternative communication on the communicative effectiveness of an individual with a progressive language disorder. *International Journal of Rehabilitation Research*, 29(2): 151–153. (AAC for people with PPA.)

Petheram, B. (Ed.). (2015). *Computers and Aphasia: A Special Issue of* Aphasiology. Psychology Press.

Pierce, J. E., O'Halloran, R., Togher, L., Nickels, L., Copland, D., Godecke, E., Meinzer, M., Rai, T., Cadilhac, D. A., Kim, J., Hurley, M., Foster, A., Carragher, M., Wilcox, C., Steel, G., & Rose, M. L. (2023) Acceptability, feasibility and preliminary efficacy of low-moderate intensity CIAT-Plus and M-MAT in chronic aphasia after stroke. *Topics in Stroke Rehabilitation*, 31(1): 44–56.

Poirier, S. È., Fossard, M., & Monetta. L. (2021). The efficacy of treatments for sentence production deficits in aphasia: a systematic review. *Aphasiology*, 37(1): 122–142. https://doi.org/10.1080/02687038.2021.1983152

Purdy, M., & Koch, A. (2006). Prediction of strategy usage by adults with aphasia. *Aphasiology*, 20(2–4): 337–348. https://doi.org/10.1080/02687030500475085

Raymer, A. M., & Roitsch, J. (2022). Word retrieval treatments in aphasia: a survey of professional practice. *Aphasiology*, 37(7): 954–979. https://doi.org/10.1080/02687038.2022.2063791

Rose, M. L., Nickels, L., Copland, D., Togher, L., Godecke, E., Meinzer, M., Rai, T., Cadilhac, D. A., Kim, J., Hurley, M., Foster, A., Carragher, M., Wilcox, C., Pierce, J. E., & Steel, G. (2022). Results of the COMPARE trial of constraint-induced or multimodality aphasia therapy compared with usual care in chronic post-stroke aphasia. *Journal of Neurology, Neurosurgery & Psychiatry*, 93(6): 573–581.

Rose, M. L., Raymer, A. M., Lanyon, L. E., & Attard, M. C. (2013). A systematic review of gesture treatments for post-stroke aphasia. *Aphasiology*, 27(9): 1090–1127. doi:10.1080/02687038.2013.826473

Russo, M. J., Prodan, V., Meda, N. N., Carcavallo, L., Muracioli, A., Sabe, L., Bonamico, L., Allegri, R. F., & Olmos, L. (2017). High-technology augmentative communication for adults with post-stroke aphasia: a systematic review. *Expert Review of Medical Devices*, 14(5): 355–370. https://doi.org/10.1080/17434440.2017.1324291

Schwartz, M., Saffran, E., Fink, R., Myers, J. & Martin, N. (1994) Mapping therapy: a treatment programme for agrammatism. *Aphasiology*, 8(1): 19–54. https://doi.org/10.1080/02687039408248639

Shenoy, R., Harvey, S., Krishnan, G., & Nickels, L. (2024). Sorting the "mixed bag" of semantic tasks in aphasia therapy: a scoping review. *Aphasiology*, 1–38. https://doi.org/10.1080/02687038.2024.2401421

Simmons-Mackie, N., & Kagan, A. (2022). *Measure of Supported Conversation & Behavior Change (MSCBC)*. Aphasia Institute, Toronto, ON. https://www.aphasia.ca/VF_MSCBC

Simmons-Mackie, N., King, J. M., & Beukelman, D. R. (2013) *Supporting Communication for Adults with Acute and Chronic Aphasia*. Brookes Publishing. (Excerpt communication-support-for-everyday-life-situations.pdf)

Simmons-Mackie, N., King, J. M., & Beukelman, D. R. Felson Duchan, J. & Byng, S. (Eds.).. (2004). Challenging aphasia therapies: broadening the discourse and extending the boundaries. Taylor & Francis.

Simmons-Mackie, N., Raymer, A., Cherney, L. R. (2016). Communication partner training in aphasia: an updated systematic review. *Archives of Physical Medicine and Rehabilitation*, 97(12): 2202–2221.

Slobin, D. (1996). From 'thought and language' to 'thinking for speaking'. In J. Gumperz & S. Levinson (Eds.), *Rethinking Linguistic Relativity* (pp. 70–96). Cambridge University Press.

Sze, W. P., Hameau, S., Warren, J., & Best, W. (2020). Identifying the components of a successful spoken naming therapy: a meta-analysis of word-finding interventions for adults with aphasia. *Aphasiology*, 35(1): 33–72. https://doi.org/10.1080/02687038.2020.1781419

van Nispen, K., Mieke, W., van de Sandt-Koenderman, E., & Krahmer, E. (2018). The comprehensibility of pantomimes produced by people with aphasia. *International Journal of Language & Communication Disorders*, 53: 85–100. https://doi.org/10.1111/1460-6984.12328

Whitworth, A., Webster J., & Howard, D. (2014). *A Cognitive Neuropsychological Approach to Assessment and Intervention in Aphasia: A Clinician's Guide*, 2nd ed. Psychology Press.

Wiseburn, B., & Mahoney, K. (2009). A meta-analysis of word-finding treatments for aphasia. *Aphasiology*, 23(11): 1338–1352. doi: 10.1080/02687030902732745

Chapter 10

LIVING WITH APHASIA

89 IMPACT OF APHASIA ON THE INDIVIDUAL

Aphasia has a significant negative impact on someone's quality of life, including on their relationships, ability to work, social life and ability to access services. This impact has been noted as even more negative on quality of life than cancer, Alzheimer's disease and quadriplegia (Lam & Wodchis 2010). Perhaps this should not surprise us, when we consider how so much of who we are and what we do requires communication. This negative impact affects personal identity, attitudes and feelings, as the A-FROM highlights (see Appendix 1) and you will hear about this impact of living with a language disorder from your clients and their families. People report how their lives have been turned upside down or wrecked. They are often in shock, with low mood and report feeling robbed of their lives as they knew them (see Point 95). The impact of a communication disability is often not understood by the general population, and this can mean there is a lack of support for people with aphasia and their families.

People experience living with aphasia differently, depending on such factors as life experiences, support networks, communication style, personality and their attitude, particularly how they tend to react to change and to difficult situations. In addition to the aphasia, the quality of life experienced is affected by someone's physical condition (health and mobility), by cognitive problems and by how much independence and financial stability they have, all of which have an impact on what they can do and their participation in everyday activities (Cruice et al. 2009). There will also be issues specific to the condition that caused the aphasia, e.g. ABI will have many other co-occurring problems, a brain tumour or progressive aphasia will have the issues of deterioration of functions and shortened life expectancy. Cognitive deficits can have a negative impact on self-awareness and problem-solving skills.

> Mr. A had a brain tumour, was aware of his prognosis and of the limited time he had to live. He wanted to have important conversations with loved ones, sort out his financial affairs and write letters to family and friends. He was finding his fatigue and memory problems and word finding difficulties frustrating. Mrs. A wanted to help but was not sure how, and while she was clearly distressed by the short life expectancy her husband had, she was able to focus on formulating a plan, together with Mr. A, and they worked on this in the sessions and at home. Part of the plan involved keeping a record of when Mr. A tended to feel a little brighter or had a little more energy. Then whether he could organise the conversations with family and friends around those times. He needed to find a way of telling these important people how to help him in conversation (see Point 83) including making written notes of key words and key messages he wanted to give. Doing some writing in sessions highlighted his difficulties with spelling, and he realised without prompting that he would need to think flexibly about writing letters and doing his finances. We discussed options, including dictating letters to Mrs. A, or into his phone using speech–to-text software, and discussing finances with his accountant using supported conversation, with Mrs. A leading, now she had the skills to do so. So, the SLT roles were to listen, to find out what Mr. A wanted and agree goals, to focus on what worked better/what could be successful, to suggest options and to train and empower family to broaden support for Mr. A beyond the therapy session. His time was very precious to him; I felt the pressure to make every minute of a session worthwhile and useful for him. The

> two sessions he had were full on and busy, and Mr. and Mrs. A reported that they were useful, and 'did the job' for him.

90 IMPACT OF APHASIA ON THE FAMILY

Aphasia affects the whole family, not just an individual, and the challenges faced by their partner, friends and family are usually significant. The aphasia changes the lives of those affected too; there are usually concerns about finances, the future and many changes to relationships with most people dealing with significant emotions such as loneliness, resentment, frustration, guilt and generally feeling exhausted. The family of people with aphasia experience 'third-party functioning and disability', or negative changes to their lives due to the aphasia (Grawburg et al. 2014). This includes a negative impact on their mood and well-being (Iwasaki et al. 2022) with family members of people with aphasia likely to develop depression after the onset of their family member's aphasia (Worrall et al. 2016).

Because aphasia affects communication in the family it has a significant impact on family roles and relationships. We need to provide education, support and ways to communicate. Include family members in therapy provision, welcome them to the one-to-one sessions, provide group therapy opportunities including carer support from their peers or professionals. The aphasia centre (https://theaphasiacenter.com) suggests that it is helpful to meet other people with aphasia and their families for support and advice, to remind the partner that they are not single-handedly responsible for the progress or recovery of their loved one with aphasia and do not have a magic wand, need regular breaks and time away from aphasia. Having the family able to learn about aphasia and therapy and supported conversation techniques and their commitment to being actively involved in the rehabilitation is essential to the success of the aphasia therapy. So supporting the family is an essential part of your work.

Provide training in supported conversation and psychosocial support; from yourself and from relevant services, for clients and their families (Vallury, Jones & Grey 2015). Make sure they all know about options for support. Offer to provide education about someone's aphasia and how to communicate better with them not just to the spouse, but also to the extended family, who are frequently forgotten. Where possible, also include friends in supported conversation training and in group therapy programmes (Davidson et al. 2008). Friendships can be overlooked but are often key to social participation. While some friends will offer help and support, a focus of therapy can be to have a concerted 'campaign' to engage with friends. Encourage your client and their family to do this, even though it may seem artificial and lack the spontaneity they may have enjoyed in friendships. Suggest they make a list of the people the person with aphasia would like to see. Put them in order of importance, contact the most important ones first. People may be nervous, unsure what to expect (after all, most people are unaware of what aphasia is and means). Suggest that the family prepare the friends before they meet the person with aphasia by giving them a summary of what it is, and/or a loan of a useful resource such as the *Stroke and Aphasia Handbook* (see Appendix 5). Make concrete suggestions as to what to expect and how to communicate. Have a partner or family member there to help. Reassure the friends that a little contact means a lot. Keep the visit short. Find things that this friendship may have always involved that have fewer demands on communication (going for a walk, watching a film together, listening to music, going for a coffee, looking at photos, crafts and making things, gardening).

91 LIVING WELL WITH APHASIA

There is the idea of adapting or adjusting to aphasia or accepting it. What adaptation or adjustment or acceptance might mean to each person with aphasia and their family will vary

(Brown et al. 2011). The idea of being in harmony with oneself is a useful approach. It implies an acceptance of the current situation brought on by a chronic condition, which involves hope, courage and an engagement in life as it now is. The hope may be for improvement, in the aphasia and/or in managing to communicate more easily despite the aphasia. Without some hope and engagement in life, there can be despondency and despair (Delmar et al. 2005). Ideally, there is a balance of acceptance and the motivation that hope brings.

There are positive adaptive processes that we see in people living successfully with aphasia. These are often related not only to communication issues but also to meaningful relationships, being engaged in activities or aiming to live positively (Brown et al. 2010). Factors that contribute to living well with aphasia include psychological factors, the absence of or successful treatment of any depression and anxiety (see Points 96 and 99) and someone's previous personality traits and psychological resources. Important positive ones include self-awareness, confidence and the ability to cope. Someone who had previous strategies for managing difficulties, such as exercise, yoga or meditation can look to some of these, perhaps in adapted forms. Practical issues that contribute include financial stability (DuBay et al. 2011) and the support someone gets from relationships and their social network (Worrall et al. 2017).

You will see many positive examples of people living well with aphasia. One client wanted to inspire other people with aphasia not to give up. He continued to be out in the world, communicating as best he could. He reported that when he was on holiday in Egypt and trying to talk to the tour guide, his word retrieval difficulties were obvious. He did not let that stop him talking and used self-disclosure to manage the awkwardness of the situation, telling the guide about his aphasia. The tour guide's father had also had a stroke and he took my client home, where he enjoyed an impromptu, international aphasia support group meeting. Following a stroke, Debra Myerson had significant aphasia. In her book (Myerson 2019), she describes how for her, the loss of her previous life with its roles, relationships and identity was devastating.

> Understanding and accepting the loss of my old life was one of the hardest parts of my recovery and rebuilding process ... I've spent the past eight years working to regain my sense of self, trying to answer the question: who am I now?

She describes the process of grieving what she had lost and beginning to look forward.

92 A THERAPY GOAL

Addressing the impact of the aphasia on someone also involves understanding more about that person, how and where they want to use their speech and language and how their participation in the things they want to do has been or might be affected by the aphasia. This can mean that alongside therapy to maximise recovery of language, a therapy goal is to promote communicating as well as possible with the speech and language available (using supported conversation) and addressing how to communicate in order to participate in their everyday lives. Since living well with something that is chronic and changes benefits from ongoing support, the importance of helping people to access support from aphasia organisations and charities is clear.

93 ADAPTING THE ENVIRONMENT

Beyond the clinic, we are aware of a lack of understanding of aphasia in the wider world, which means that people with aphasia face barriers to participating in work and social activities because of their aphasia. Challenging the barriers to communication is an enormous task. As SLTs we can do this in small ways by providing aphasia-friendly information and training in supported conversation to our clients and their families and friends. We can do this in the places we work, e.g. hospitals or residential homes. Looking for ways to connect people with aphasia with their communities can increase confidence and social engagement and educate the wider world about aphasia. We can advertise, promote and support aphasia organisations and community aphasia groups (see useful links in Appendix 5). Help your clients look for opportunities to participate in social activities including those where the demand on language is reduced; these are sometimes designed for people with aphasia (Pieri et al. 2023).

94 PUBLIC AWARENESS OF APHASIA

Barriers to communication start with a lack of awareness of aphasia in the general public. In an international survey (Simmons-Mackie et al. 2002) only 13.6 per cent of respondents said they had heard of aphasia and only 5.4 per cent had some basic knowledge of what it was. Another survey across several continents (Code et al. 2016) 37 per cent had heard of aphasia with 9 per cent having basic knowledge of what it is. It is important to note that 99 per cent of respondents had heard of a stroke and 53 per cent had a basic knowledge of it, 96 per cent of Parkinson's disease and 31 per cent had a basic knowledge of it. Why does that matter? In general, support from people around us matters when we are dealing with significant health issues or changes in our lives. When no one has heard of the difficulties we are dealing with, it is more difficult for them to offer appropriate support. Sometimes the lack of understanding leads to stigma and avoidance. People with aphasia may be seen by some as having some kind of mental breakdown or dementia. The loss of a basic function such as language is a frightening prospect for most people. These reactions and lack of support can mean that the feelings of isolation increase which contribute further to the social withdrawal that a communication difficulty causes anyway. People with aphasia may lose their friends (Manning et al. 2021). This in turn can lead to anxiety and depression (see Points 95 and 96). Lack of understanding in the world around someone with aphasia can mean that people either are, or feel, unaccepted in the public sphere, particularly in the workplace.

When people with aphasia try to access services, this lack of understanding of what aphasia is and of how to support them to communicate can also affect the quality of services they receive. In terms of mental health services, ignorance of aphasia can lead to inappropriate referrals and inadequate treatment (see Point 99). People affected by aphasia have difficulty in interacting with doctors and other service providers who often do not know how to support communication or provide information in an accessible way. There is a need to recognise that people with aphasia must have their communication requirements met, with the equivalent of interpreters, with supported conversation training across the health sector. Not to do so discriminates against them. There is some recognition of the need for some health care professionals to recognise and screen for aphasia (O'Sullivan, Brownsett & Copland 2019) but not nearly enough training takes place in hospitals, GP surgeries, post offices or buses – everywhere that someone with aphasia might want to go and be able to communicate.

Take part in public campaigns, such as the aphasia awareness months promoted by aphasia organisations. They are an opportunity to contact the local and national media with human-interest stories, offer to give a talk in your local community or put up posters. Involve your clients with aphasia in the campaigns. In all the education about aphasia, include a focus on the barriers to someone with aphasia participating in their lives, giving people clear and practical suggestions about how to enable better conversations.

People with aphasia know how important it is to keep communicating, to keep trying despite the difficulties. And they know what a difference it makes when the responses of people they meet to their aphasia is helpful. As one client described:

My name is Steve
  I'm 52 now.
  I had aphasia ... 4 years ago
  I couldn't say any words ... couldn't say language ... not numbers!
  I'm moving ... getting better ... but it's hard ... difficult.

> **Some people are so nice ... helpful ... so(me) people don't listen ...**
>
> **When I'm saying things ... slowly ... some people will talk something else ... different ... to stop me ... but frustrating.** I need to say more things ... restaurants ... coffee ... bar.
>
> Helps me to say words and talk

95 THE PSYCHOLOGICAL IMPACT OF APHASIA

The 'Personal Identity, Attitudes and Feelings' part of the A-FROM (see Appendix 1) highlight the changes that aphasia brings not only to communication but also to someone's psychological health (Kagan et al. 2008). Changes result from both physiological and psychological factors.

96 THE PHYSIOLOGICAL AND PSYCHOLOGICAL FACTORS

It is likely that the brain lesion itself disrupts mood regulation (De Ryck et al. 2014) and you may see emotional lability with involuntary laughing or crying. The severity but not the type of stroke may increase the likelihood of depression. Fatigue and physical pain are two physiological factors that have a negative influence on someone's ability to concentrate, focus, process language and engage in rehabilitation.

Having a stroke, brain injury or diagnosis of a brain tumour are all traumatic events, leading to grief and loss in response to the sudden changes/loss of their usual abilities. A brain lesion may cause paralysis, loss of mobility and independent living. The loss of independence can lead to low mood, low self-esteem and irritability. The aphasia involves a sudden loss of language function and ability to communicate. With this comes the loss of independence, relationships, jobs and hobbies. Loss of language produces a grief reaction equivalent to that experienced by those who have suffered the death of a loved one (Jackson 1988). Language is so essential to being human that the impairment of communication skills after a stroke can lead to higher-than-normal levels of frustration, stress, hopelessness, depression and anxiety. Aphasia could be described as a 'disorder of the person' as well as a disorder of language (Sarno 1993). And because aphasia by its nature makes interacting with others difficult, it can lead to feelings of isolation, inferiority, embarrassment and shame. Some people with aphasia report an existential loneliness; a profound separateness from who they used to be, from other people and from the world.

DEPRESSION

The prevalence of depression after stroke is approximately 31 per cent (Hackett et al. 2014); but 70 per cent in people with aphasia in the first three months post stroke (De Wit et al. 2008). People with post-stroke depression are less likely to show improvements in functions and to return to their previous life activities, with poor quality of life outcomes. Post-stroke depression might itself affect cognitive processing, especially executive dysfunction (Robinson & Spalletta 2010) which in turn affects language and conversation, and the ability to engage with aphasia therapy.

ANXIETY

The proportion of people with significant anxiety after stroke is between 18 and 25 per cent (Campbell Burton et al. 2013). Anxiety is observed in perhaps 44 per cent of people with aphasia, with the risk factors for anxiety appearing to be the severity of the aphasia and younger age (Morris et al. 2017). People with aphasia report feeling anxious about having another stroke, about not being able to communicate and about being a burden to their family and friends. You may see 'linguistic anxiety' (Cahana-Amitay et al. 2011), anticipating errors and failure to communicate and feelings of embarrassment. People then avoid social situations where they will need to communicate. This leads to further isolation from other people and increased loneliness.

97 ADDRESSING PSYCHOLOGICAL ISSUES

Psychological issues can have a significant impact on the ability to engage with therapy (Baker et al. 2020) and live better with the aphasia (Cruice, Worrall and Hickson 2011). Take them into account during assessment (see Point 35 and Appendix 4 for examples of relevant assessments). Ask what is being done to address any low mood, either on the ward or via a GP. Low mood should not preclude you from offering therapy; but find out where to refer on for appropriate psychological support. What you say – or don't say – in therapy sessions can be helpful – or unhelpful. Remember to observe. Notice whether the client and/or their family members express or exhibit any distress, anger, anxiety or frustration in their facial expressions, in their posture.

ASK QUESTIONS

Start to find out how someone with aphasia and their family are finding life after the stroke or head injury. 'Tell me why you are here' or 'Tell me what happened'. Find out what the person with aphasia and their family report about changes in mood, about how they are feeling generally. Ask a general question: 'How are you getting on?' or 'How are you feeling?' or 'What can I help with?' can give you your first glimpse of where the people in front of you are in terms of their mood. Do they report or exhibit anxiety or distress, anger or frustration? Do they use the words 'worried', 'sad', 'concerned'', 'angry', 'upset' or 'frustrated'? Or do they hint at these emotions with understatements such as, 'not feeling great', 'it's a bit difficult'?

Note the language and speech production in the answers or attempts at answers of the client and their family. If you have asked about the event that brought about the aphasia, one of the most important narratives you will hear in this client's therapy with you, the story may be expressed via tears and fits of rage rather than words. The client may get angry, shout about what has happened, about the medical care or experience in hospital, about the huge changes in their lives. A person with no speech can still bang on the door, throw papers off the table, wave their hands in your face. As long as you do not feel physically under threat (see Point 100) try to tolerate this behaviour as the only way that person can express themselves at that moment. How you respond to this key story is important; listening, paraphrasing, reflecting and questioning what you hear from both the person with aphasia and their family. Choosing not to ask more questions about something said is also important. **Listen** more than you speak. Pay careful attention to what is being said. Make eye contact to indicate that you are listening. Don't judge what you hear. Don't interrupt. Listen for longer than you might think is necessary, sit in the silence and wait. When you work with people with aphasia you will wait a lot while someone navigates their word retrieval difficulties, for example, or their sentence processing problems. Provide a model to the family of the person with aphasia of listening; how to listen for longer than usual, how to wait and begin to model supported conversation techniques. Create an atmosphere in the therapy sessions where difficult emotions such as frustration and despair and loss are accepted as part of the consequences of aphasia and can be expressed by the person with aphasia and their family. Be prepared and willing to engage in more challenging or what are usefully referred to as 'tender' conversations (Manix 2021). Sessions can then be places where aphasia therapy includes both the difficult emotions and where there is support and hope.

Be clear with yourself and your clients what your professional limitations are in terms of what you can offer in terms of psychological support. Unless you have had further specific training, you are not a counsellor or psychotherapist, nor are you a couples' therapist/marriage guidance counsellor or family therapist. Learn to recognise when you are drawn into conversations or situations where the issues go beyond your professional remit. Know where to refer for psychological support. You do not have to provide the answers. But if you are going to ask someone to reveal how they are feeling, you must make sure that you are genuinely able to sit with and tolerate expressions of emotion and know what may be needed from you (see Point 100). Don't be surprised if you have reactions to the emotions you hear. SLTs normally receive training in safeguarding; including knowing that if a client expresses a plan or desire to kill themselves, there is a professional responsibility to report this to their medical team; to the consultant or senior medical staff or to their GP and, of course, to any psychologist or counsellor they are seeing. In the community, as well as the GP surgery, there may be local, emergency mental health teams you can contact to make sure that other parts of the health system are aware of your concerns about your client.

> Mr. R was in his 40s and often visibly distressed by the almost complete loss of his speech and of his ability to work. He used gestures, facial expressions and pointed to a route on a map to carefully outline his plan to drive to the nearby river and drive into the water, in order to kill himself. While it was difficult for him to drive, it was not impossible. After the session, I contacted his GP to tell him about Mr. R's low mood and clear intention to harm himself. The GP saw Mr. R and prescribed antidepressants. I continued to see Mr. R for treatment of his aphasia, and he engaged in therapy well, including regular home practice and involvement of his whole family in his rehabilitation.
>
> Mr. N was angry and frustrated by his aphasia and its enormous, negative impact on his life. In one session he used accurate gestures to show that he was going to shoot himself. As he lived in the countryside, with access to guns, this was not an empty threat. The information was reported to Mr. N's GP who took on responsibility for the situation with referrals for psychological assessment and support.

SLTs do not routinely get training in counselling but often learn basic counselling skills as part of their qualifications. SLTs also learn these skills on clinical placements, from discussions with colleagues (other SLTs, or clinical psychologists or occupational therapists, for example) and perhaps their own psychological therapy/counselling. You will find it essential to distinguish between having counselling skills and providing counselling, and learn about key areas such as developing the therapeutic relationship, setting boundaries, knowing ways of responding, self-disclosure and loss. It can be helpful to understand the stages of grief and bereavement. This will have an impact on how you manage the ending of therapy (see Point 24).

Understanding what has happened and normalising the impact on well-being has been shown to be helpful. Education about brain injury is carried out in groups at the Wolfson Neurorehabilitation Centre, including working on reconstructing identity (James 2011). Aphasia can be experienced as "identity theft" (Shadden 2005). Rebuilding personal identity can be an important part of someone learning to live well with aphasia. Normalise the feelings the client and their family express by using key words openly, for example, 'most people with aphasia feel sad/very sad/very low/depressed/anxious/frustrated'; try different words out and notice what response they produce, if any.

Suggest information and facts to give their friends and family; explaining what aphasia is and its effects, clarifying that having aphasia does not mean that you cannot think for yourself, but that it is difficult for you to express those thoughts.
. Aphasia is a language problem that masks a person's inherent competence, 'I know that you know' (Kagan 1995) Provide reassurance: while you may be experiencing low mood, be upset and anxious about what has happened, you are still a competent adult. You have not lost your intellect. You have not lost your mind. You still have your thoughts and ideas. Aphasia means it is difficult for you to express those thoughts. Your thoughts and your words are disconnected. Therapy aims to reconnect them.

Provide Education about the risks of the loss of social life and friends and aim to reduce isolation early in the rehabilitation process. Suggest what they can do to try and deal with this; phrase this in terms of: it is very common for friends and family to find it difficult to know how to respond to what has happened and how to have a conversation with you. Reassure them that people with aphasia do report feeling worried about other people's perceptions and expectations.

Provide education about other physical or cognitive issues that have an impact on communication, e.g. fatigue. This can help someone to appreciate that their difficulties with communication are normal, complex and involve more than the aphasia itself; so that rather than feeling incompetent they can plan to compensate for the many issues they are dealing with. This way, someone may be encouraged to monitor their level of fatigue, put regular breaks in place during the day and plan when to have conversations in advance.

98 ASSESSMENT OF WELL-BEING

At assessment you should also ask about the client's psychological or psychiatric history; any previous history of depression or anxiety may predispose someone to further episodes. Asking about someone's personality traits prior to the aphasia is useful because how someone may manage the impact of the aphasia on their lives is likely to be influenced by pre-existing personality. Many services will have developed questionnaires about the person with aphasia for the family or spouse to complete, often while on the ward. These ask questions about someone's previous job, family background, languages spoken and hobbies and also asks for descriptions of the person in terms of their usual behaviour ('Is he usually cheerful/a bit of a worrier?', for example). You can use these descriptions as a starting point. How accurate these descriptions are will depend on the type and level of relationship between the person with aphasia and whoever completes the questionnaire.

The A-FROM aspect of 'Personal Identity, Attitudes and Feelings' (see Appendix 1) provides a useful set of headings, which includes 'Feelings' and 'Your view of yourself'. The social model highlights aphasia as a communication disability and it may be one aspect of your therapy provision to address this. Using the word 'disability' will depend on each client; is it a word they use? It might be helpful with people who spend a lot of time and energy concealing word retrieval difficulties, for example (see 'linguistic anxiety' Point 96). You could use the iceberg metaphor (often used with people who stammer) to discuss both the obvious and the hidden aspects of aphasia which affect someone's abilities and confidence. The word retrieval difficulties with the long pauses in conversations and the word errors are seen by the listener, the embarrassment, tension and avoidance of words and situations is hidden like the iceberg under the water (Sheehan 1958).

> A client with cognitive-communication difficulties after ABI (a result of a head injury sustained in a road traffic accident) had made a lot of progress in his communication and said that because he was doing so well, the difficulties he was having were unseen and belittled by others (he was told, 'Oh, you're back to normal now'). He certainly wanted to be seen as the person he was before the accident and not viewed as different. However, he was aware that on returning to work he would have some issues with group conversations, with multitasking, with some word retrieval difficulties, missing information that people tell him in conversation and was aware of feeling anxious about all these. How would people react to the overt difficulties: with word retrieval (the silences, the word errors) to his leaving the room when there were too many people talking for him to manage, to him asking for repetition of information? They wouldn't see the hidden (covert) difficulties, particularly the negative emotions he experienced, of fear, embarrassment, shame or humiliation. Therapy included identifying the overt and covert issues. In particular, looking at how the covert

> issues lead to changes in his behaviour, particularly that in trying to hide the difficulties with word retrieval, etc. he was avoiding words, conversations, speaking to people, avoiding certain situations (groups, telephone calls) and relationships and how this avoidance could affect his ability to do the things he wanted to do, such as his job.

99 PSYCHOLOGICAL TREATMENTS, SUPPORT AND DEVELOPING STRATEGIES

Many SLTs do not feel confident about addressing the psychological issues of their clients (Northcott et al. 2017). While the SLT may have training and/or clinical experience that gives them some basic counselling skills, there are often situations where the person with aphasia and/or their family members need more skilled, professional psychological or psychiatric support or help. You may already be working in an environment such as a Mental Health Trust where clients are referred with co-existing mental health diagnoses. Your client may present with pre-existing psychological or psychiatric issues. It is important to know when you do not have the psychological training to manage some emotional states. You could seek further training in managing these, for example, the CLEAR: Counselling Education in Aphasia Rehabilitation programme(Shafer, Haley & Jacks 2023). You may want to discuss psychological issues that arise with clients with your colleagues, usually clinical psychologists, psychiatrists, nurses and occupational therapists. It is helpful to learn more about a client's psychological profile or disorders from colleagues with more knowledge and experience. Their diagnoses and/or advice can help guide your therapy interactions and expectations; both of yourself and of your client. In some cases, you may be advised that someone's psychological profile makes success in therapy difficult for you to achieve. This can be helpful in guiding your expectations and management. Make sure you know how and where to refer clients within your organisation and to other support networks where appropriate (see Appendix 5).

PSYCHIATRY

You could discuss referrals with your client's GP or doctors on the ward. There is evidence that the use of antidepressants is helpful for treating post-stroke anxiety as well as leading to improved cognitive function (Starkstein, Mizrahi and Power 2008, Mitchell et al.2009).

PSYCHOLOGY

There is evidence that behavioural therapy may improve the mood of people with aphasia (Thomas et al. 2013) and the use of psychotherapy can be helpful for treating post-stroke anxiety (Mikolajczyk & Bateman 2012). However, having aphasia makes it more difficult to ask for and receive help. People with aphasia often do not get accurate diagnoses of a mood disorder or mental health condition and as a result, do not have access to mental health services (Simmons-Mackie & Damico 2007). 'Talking therapies' by their very nature rely on someone being able to understand what is said to them by the therapist/counsellor and then verbalise their thoughts. Someone with aphasia is likely to find it difficult to both understand the language used by a counsellor and express their thoughts and emotions using the spoken word, if at all. However, there are people who can adapt their counselling or psychological therapy to be accessible to people with aphasia. Some therapies are less reliant on a high level of communication abilities, or modify the communication demands to make the support accessible for people with aphasia, such as art therapy (Andrew 2015) and music therapy (Gadberry & Ramachandra 2015). Other techniques involve learning self-regulation strategies (Pieri et al. 2023) and include mind-body practices such as meditation and mindfulness (Yeates 2019).

MINDFULNESS AND MEDITATION

Kabat-Zinn (1994) describes mindfulness as purposefully paying attention to the present moment, without judgement. Some aspects of a mindfulness programme may be effective in reducing anxiety in people with aphasia (Dickinson, Friary and McCann 2017). Mindfulness based stress reduction (MBSR) courses teach self-management of symptoms of anxiety and depression via meditation and mindfulness breathing. The instructions and ideas can involve language that is challenging for people with aphasia to understand. There is potential for people with aphasia to use modified mindfulness courses (HEADS: UP Aphasia Helping Ease Anxiety and Depression Following Stroke, UK Stroke Association 2019–2023). One appealing aspect of mindfulness and meditation for people with aphasia is that the focus of mindfulness meditation is on *being* as you are, without judgement: rather than doing and achieving. This can provide a welcome contrast to the demands of rehabilitation.

100 LOOKING AFTER YOURSELF: SUPPORT AND DEVELOPMENT

Spending time with people who are going through traumatic events and who may be depressed or anxious is probably an inevitable consequence of working with people with aphasia and is likely to have an impact on you. Learning how best to manage that impact and maintain your own equilibrium is an important part of being a good clinician. Part of your development as an aphasia therapist is to learn to offer acceptance of these emotions in the clinic, by being with the person and their emotions. Part of it is also to understand yourself better. How do you react? Are you very uncomfortable when emotions are expressed? How do you increase your capacity to recognise what is (or is not) appropriate or necessary and what skills might you need to develop?

The Health Care and Professions Council (HCPC) standards of proficiency for SLTs include looking after our own health and well-being. This includes identifying any anxiety and stress in ourselves and recognising the potential impact on our practice, seeking help and support when necessary. Your anxieties may also be to do with your own life issues and/or pressures of the amount and/or complexity of your workload.

TALK ABOUT YOUR WORK

You may find it helpful to talk about your work, about what goes well and is successful as well as what is challenging or difficult. Talking about it can help to clarify your thoughts and to recognise the impact of the work on you as a clinician and as a person. Always preserve the confidentiality of your client, their family and friends when you talk about them; use terms like, 'Mr. A'.

With colleagues: Sometimes these discussions can constitute 'peer supervision'; giving you an opportunity to check your knowledge about the client's aphasia and to discuss possible assessment and therapy options. You may be able to talk about what is challenging about the client and/or their family. Resist the temptation to 'bad-mouth' your clients or to resort to laughing at them and their situation; 'black humour' is sometimes seen as a coping mechanism in health care, particularly when clients have been through distressing accidents causing head injuries or are dying of a brain tumour, but it rarely provides real comfort and tends to belittle our humanity.

With a clinical supervisor: Access clinical supervision where it is available; this may be provided by another SLT (in your health care trust or independently), usually experienced clinicians who have had specific training in providing confidential, structured opportunities for the SLT to be supported to explore personal and professional issues relating to work. They may/may not have knowledge and experience of working with aphasia. An important aspect of clinical supervision is to be ready to accept feedback and suggestions of how to improve. Don't just look for support from your supervisor; be ready to be challenged about your thinking and your work.

With friends and family: Again this must be done preserving client confidentiality. If friends and family work in education, psychology or medicine they will probably be able to relate to some of the issues you describe. Be open to learning from everyone you talk to; they may have a different way of thinking about the issue which can give you another approach.

With a therapist: Clinical supervision is not counselling or therapy, and there may be times when you would find it useful to see a counsellor or psychotherapist yourself, someone who can help you develop as a person and as a clinician. It may be a good idea to consider therapy when you find that you are noticing particular reactions to clients, families or situations and a pattern of thoughts/feelings emerging that trouble you or get in the way of your life, including your work.

REFERENCES

Andrew, C. (2015). Drawing for people with aphasia: an investigation into the possible benefits of learning observational drawing for people with aphasia. Masters dissertation, City University London.

Baker, C., Worrall, L., Rose, M., & Ryan, B. (2020). 'It was really dark': the experiences and preferences of people with aphasia to manage mood changes and depression. *Aphasiology*, 34(1): 19–46. doi:10.1080/02687038.2019.1673304

Brown, K., Worrall, L., Davidson, B., & Howe, T. (2010). Snapshots of success: an insider perspective on living successfully with aphasia. *Aphasiology*, 24(10): 1267–1295. https://doi.org/10.1080/02687031003755429

Brown, K., Worrall, L., Davidson, B., & Howe, T. (2011). Living successfully with aphasia: family members share their views. *Topics in Stroke Rehabilitation*, 18(5): 536–548. https://doi.org/10.1310/tsr1805-536

Cahana-Amitay, D., et al. (2011). Language as a stressor in aphasia. *Aphasiology*, 25, 593–614.

Campbell Burton, C. A., Murray, J., Holmes, J., Astin, F., Greenwood, D., Knapp, P. (2013). Frequency of anxiety after stroke: a systematic review and meta-analysis of observational studies. *International Journal of Stroke*, 8(7): 545–559. doi: 10.1111/j.1747-4949.2012.00906

Code, C., Papathanasiou, I., Rubio-Bruno, S., Cabana, M. de L., Villanueva, M. M., Haaland-Johansen, L., Prizl-Jakovac, T., Leko, A., Zemva, N., Patterson, R., Berry, R., Rochon, E., Leonard, C., & Robert, A. (2016). International patterns of the public awareness of aphasia. *International Journal of Language and Communication Disorders*, 51(3): 276–284. doi: 10.1111/1460-6984.12204

Cruice, M., Worrall, L., Hickson, L., & Murison, R. (2003). Finding a focus for quality of life with aphasia: social and emotional health, and psychological well-being. *Aphasiology*, 17(4): 333–353. doi: https://doi.org/10.1080/02687030244000707

Cruice, M., Worrall, L., & Hickson, L. (2006). Quantifying aphasic people's social lives in the context of non-aphasic peers. *Aphasiology*, 20(12): 1210–1225. doi: 10.1080/02687030600790136

Cruice, M., Worrall, L., & Hickson, L. (2011). Reporting on psychological well-being of older adults with chronic aphasia in the context of unaffected peers. *Disability and Rehabilitation*, 33(3), 219–228. https://doi.org/10.3109/09638288.2010.503835

Davidson, B., Howe, T., Worrall, L., Hickson, L., & Togher, L. (2008). Social participation for older people with aphasia: the impact of communication disability on friendships. *Topics in Stroke Rehabilitation*, 15(4): 325–340. doi: 10.1310/tsr1504-325

Delmar, C., Bøje, T., Dylmer, D., Forup, L., Jakobsen, C., Møller, M., Sønder, H., & Pedersen, B. D. (2005). Achieving harmony with oneself: life with a chronic illness. *Scandinavian Journal of Caring Sciences*, 19(3): 204–212. https://doi.org/10.1111/j.1471-6712.2005.00334.x

De Ryck, A., Fransen, E., Brouns, R., Geurden, M., Peij, D., Mariën, P., De Deyn, P. P., & Engelborghs, S. (2014). Poststroke depression and its multifactorial nature: results from a prospective longitudinal study. *Journal of the Neurological Sciences*, 347(1–2): 159–-166. https://doi.org/10.1016/j.jns.2014.09.038

De Wit, L., Putman, K., Baert, I., Lincoln, N. B., Angst, F., Beyens, H., Bogaerts, K., Brinkmann, N., Connell, L., Dejaeger, E., De Weerdt, W,, Jenni, W., Kaske, C., Komarek, A., Lesaffre, E., Leys, M., Louckx, F., Schuback, B., Schupp, W., Smith, B., & Feys, H. (2008). Anxiety and depression in the first six months after stroke: a longitudinal multicentre study. *Disability and Rehabilitation*, 30(24):1858–1866. doi:10.1080/09638280701708736

Dickinson, J., Friary, P., & McCann, C. M. (2017). The influence of mindfulness meditation on communication and anxiety: a case study of a person with aphasia. *Aphasiology*, 31(9): 1044–1058. doi: 10.1080/02687038.2016.1234582

DuBay, M. F., Laures-Gore, J. S., Matheny, K., & Romski, M. A. (2011). Coping resources in individuals with aphasia. *Aphasiology*, 25(9): 1016–1029. https://doi.org/10.1080/02687038.2011.570933

Gadberry, A. L., & Ramachandra, V. (2015). The effectiveness of a music therapy protocol for a person with nonfluent aphasia: a preliminary case report. *Music and Medicine*, 7(1): 46–48. https://doi.org/10.47513/mmd.v7i1.297

Grawburg, M., Howe, T., Worrall, L, & Scarinci, N. (2014). Describing the impact of aphasia on close family members using the ICF framework. *Disability and Rehabilitation*, 36(14): 1184–1195. doi: 10.3109/09638288.2013.834984.

Hackett, M. L., Yapa, C., Parag, V., & Anderson, C. S. (2005). Frequency of depression after stroke: a systematic review of observational studies. *Stroke*, 36(6): 1330-1340. doi: 10.1161/01.STR.0000165928.19135.3

Hilari, K., & Botting, B. (Eds.) (2021). *The Impact of Communication Disability Across the Lifespan*. J&R Press.

James, K. (2011). *The Strands of Speech and Language Therapy: Weaving Plan for Neurorehabilitation*, 1st ed. Routledge. https://doi.org/10.4324/9781003072461

Kabat-Zinn, J. (1994). *Wherever You Go, There You Are. Mindfulness Meditation in Everyday Life*. New Hyperion.

Kagan, A. (1995). Revealing the competence of aphasic adults through conversation: a challenge to health professionals. *Topics in Stroke Rehabilitation*, 2: 15–28.

Kagan, A., Simmons-Mackie, N., Rowland, A., Huijbregts, M., Shumway, E., McEwen, S., Threats, T., & Sharp, S. (2008). Counting what counts: a framework for capturing real-life outcomes of aphasia intervention. *Aphasiology*, 22(3): 258–280. https://doi.org/10.1080/02687030701282595

Lam, J. M., & Wodchis, W. P. (2010). The relationship of 60 disease diagnoses and 15 conditions to preference-based health-related quality of life in Ontario hospital-based long-term care residents. *Medical Care*, 484(4): 380–387. doi: 10.1097/MLR.0b013e3181ca2647

Manning, M., MacFarlane, A., Hickey, A., Galvin, R., & Franklin, S. (2021). 'I hated being ghosted' – The relevance of social participation for living well with post-stroke aphasia: qualitative interviews with working aged adults. *Health Expectations*, 24(4): 1504–1515. https://doi.org/10.1111/hex. 13291

Mannix, K. (2021). *Listen: How to Find the Words for Tender Conversations*. William Collins.

Mikolajczyk, A., & Bateman, A. (2012). Psychodynamic counselling after stroke: a pilot service development project and evaluation. *Advances in Clinical Neuroscience and Rehabilitation* https://doi.org/10.47795/KNIF1633

Mitchell, P., Veith, R., Becker, K., Buzaitis, A., Cain, K., Fruin, M., Tirschwell, D., & Teri, L. (2009). Brief psychosocial-behavioral intervention with antidepressant reduces poststroke depression significantly more than usual care with antidepressant. *Stroke*, 40(9): 3073–3078.

Morris, R., Eccles, A., Ryan, B., & Kneebone, I. (2017). Prevalence of anxiety in people with aphasia after stroke, *Aphasiology*, 31(12): 1410–1415. doi: 10.1080/02687038.2017.1304633

Myerson, D. (2019). *Identity Theft*. Andrews McMeel Publishing.

Northcott, S., Simpson, A., Simpson, A., Moss, B., Ahmed, N., & Hilari, K. (2017). How do speech and language therapists address the psychosocial well-being of people with aphasia? Results of a UK on-line survey. *International Journal of Language and Communication Disorders*, 52(3): 356–373. doi:10.1111/1460-6984.12278

O'Sullivan, M., Brownsett, S., & Copland, D. (2019). Language and language disorders: neuroscience to clinical practice. *Practical Neurology*, 19(5): 380–388. doi:10.1136/practneurol-2018-001961

Pieri, M., Foote, H., Grealy, M., Lawrence, A., Lowit, A., & Pearl, G. (2023). Mind-body and creative arts therapies for people with aphasia: a mixed-method systematic review. *Aphasiology*, 37(3): 504–562. doi:10.1080/02687038.2022.2031862

Pound, C. (2013). An exploration of the friendship experiences of working-age adults with aphasia. PhD dissertation, Brunel University, London.

Robinson, R. G., & Spalletta, G. (2010). Poststroke depression: a review *The Canadian Journal of Psychiatry*, 55(6): 341–349.

Sarno, M. T. (1993). Aphasia rehabilitation: psychosocial and ethical considerations. *Aphasiology*, 7(4): 321–334. doi: 10.1080/02687039308249514.Shadden, B. (2005) Aphasia as identity theft: theory and practice. *Aphasiology*, 19(3–5): 211–223. doi: 10.1080/02687930444000697

Shafer, J. S., Haley, K. L., & Jacks, A. (2023) How ten speech-language pathologists provide informational counselling across the rehabilitation continuum for care partners of stroke survivors with aphasia. *Aphasiology*, 37(5): 735–760. doi: 10.1080/02687038.2022.2039371

Sheehan, J. G. (1970). Stuttering: Research and Therapy. Harper & Row.

Simmons-Mackie, N., Code, C., Armstrong, E., Stiegler, L., & Elman, R. J. (2002). What is aphasia? Results of an international survey. *Aphasiology*, 16(8): 837–848. https://doi.org/10.1080/02687030244000185

Simmons-Mackie, N. N., & Damico, J. S. (2007). Access and social inclusion in aphasia: interactional principles and applications. *Aphasiology*, 21(1): 81–97. https://doi.org/10.1080/02687030600798311

Starkstein, S., Mizrahi, R., & Power, B. (2008). Antidepressant therapy in post-stroke depression. *Expert Opinion on Pharmacotherapy*, 9(8): 1291–1298.

Swinburn, K., & Byng, D. (2006) *The Communication Disability Profile*. Connect.

Thomas, S. A., Walker, M. F., Macniven, J. A., Haworth, H., & Lincoln, N. B. (2013). Communication and low mood (CALM): a randomized controlled trial of behavioural therapy for stroke patients with aphasia. *Clinical Rehabilitation*, 27(5), 398–408.

Vallury, K. D., Jones, M., & Gray, R. (2015). Do family-oriented interventions reduce post stroke depression? A systematic review and recommendations for practice. *Topics in Stroke Rehabilitation*, 22(6):453–459. doi: 10.1179/1074935715Z.00000000061 .

Worrall, L. E, Hudson, K., Khan, A., Ryan, B., & Simmons-Mackie, N. (2017). Determinants of living well with aphasia in the first year poststroke: a prospective cohort study. *Archives of Physical Medicine and Rehabilitation*, 98(2): 235–240. doi: 10.1016/j.apmr.2016.06.020

Worrall, L., Ryan, B., Hudson, K. Kneebore, I., Simmons-Mackie, N., Khan, A., Hoffmann, T., Power, E., Togher, L., & Rose M. (2016). Reducing the psychosocial impact of aphasia on mood and quality of life in people with aphasia and the impact of caregiving in family members through the Aphasia Action Success Knowledge (Aphasia ASK) program: study protocol for a randomized controlled trial. *Trials*, 17, 153. https://doi.org/10.1186/s13063-016-1257-9

Yeates, G. N. (2019). The potential contribution of mind-body interventions within psychological support following aphasia. In K. H. Meredith and G. N. Yeates (Eds.), *Psychotherapy and Aphasia: Interventions for Emotional Wellbeing and Relationships*. Routledge.

FURTHER READING

Anderson, A. P., & Dow-Richards, C. (2014). *Aphasia Recovery Connection's Guide to Living with Aphasia*, 1st ed. CreateSpace Independent Publishing Platform.

Brumfitt, S., & Sheeran, P. (1999). *Visual Analogue Self Esteem Scale (VASES)*. Speechmark Publishing.

Brumfitt, S. M., & Sheeran, P. (1999). The development and validation of the Visual Analogue Self-Esteem Scale (VASES). *British Journal of Clinical Psychology*, 38(4): 387–400. doi: 10.1348/014466599162980

Chambers, C. (2019), *Now I Understand Aphasia*. Dog Ear Publishing. (A book for children.)

Dalton, P. (1994). *Counselling People with Communication Problems*. Sage Publications.

Greenfield, M. & Ganzfried, E. S. (2016). *Words Escape Me: Voices of Aphasia*. Balboa Press.

Hale, S. (2003). *The Man Who Lost His Language*. Penguin Books.

Jackson, H. F. (1988). Brain, cognition and grief. *Aphasiology*, 2(1): 89–92. https://doi.org/10.1080/02687038808248891

Jagoe, C., & Walsh, I. (Eds.) 2020. *Communication and Mental Health Disorders: Developing Theory, Growing Practice*. J&R Press.(This book presents recent developments in the field using a 'recovery model' principles and practices.)

Kabat-Zinn, J. (2018). *Meditation is not* What You Think. Piatkus. https://jonkabat-zinn.com and https://pressbooks.pub/app/uploads/sites/3441/2022/09/Post-Stroke-Depression_Melrose-2016.pdf (This book gives multidisciplinary perspectives on care of people with communication difficulties and mental health disorders. It explores the complex relationship between mental health and disorder, langue and communication.)

Melrose, S. (2016). Post-stroke depression: how can nurses help? *Canadian Nursing Home*, 27(1): 5–9. https://pressbooks.pub/app/uploads/sites/3441/2022/09/Post-Stroke-Depression_Melrose-2016.pdf

Mitchell, N. (2018). *After Words* (Missing collection). Amazon Original Stories. Kindle Edition. (The Missing collection comprises "six true stories about finding, restoring, or accepting the losses that define our lives." *After Words* is one woman's experience of losing and rebuilding communication after strokes.)

National Aphasia Association. (2020).*The Aphasia Caregiver Guide.* National Aphasia Association.

Panda, S., Whitworth, A., Hersh, D., & Biedermann, B. (2020). "Giving yourself some breathing room …": an exploration of group meditation for people with aphasia. *Aphasiology*, 35(12): 1544–1572. https://doi.org/10.1080/02687038.2020.1819956

UK Stroke Association. (2019–2023). HEADS: UP Aphasia, Helping Ease Anxiety and Depression following Stroke.

COUNSELLING PEOPLE WITH APHASIA

City Lit London, UK: further training: e.g. https://www.citylit.ac.uk/courses/effective-counselling-skills-for-speech-and-language-therapists

La Trobe University, Australia: CLEAR program, Counselling Education in Aphasia Rehabilitation is a short course at La Trobe University https://www.latrobe.edu.au/research/centres/health/aphasia

The Aphasia Institute, Canada: online training in how to make counselling accessible to people with aphasia through the use of SCA™ techniques. https://www.aphasia.ca/health-care-providers/education-training/training-programs-workshops

APPENDIX 1

FRAMEWORK FOR OUTCOME MEASUREMENT (A-FROM) DIAGRAM

Example:

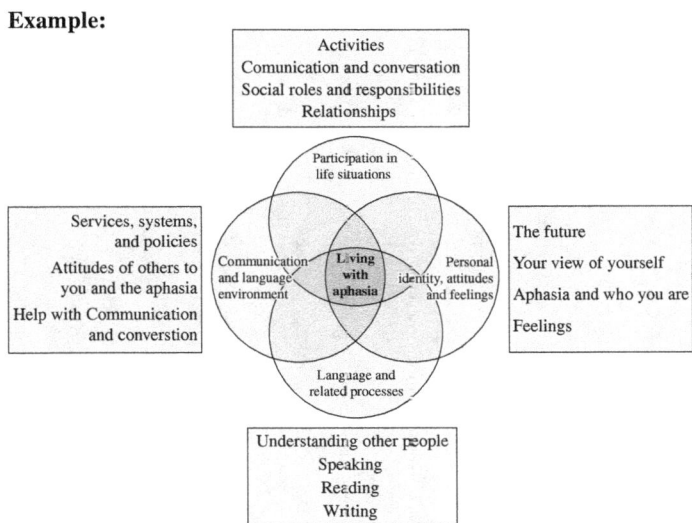

Figure 1.1 Living with aphasia: framework for outcome measurement (A-FROM) – A-FROM categories within snapshot domains

Source: Aphasia Institute, 2006; Kagan et al., 2008, p. 269.)
Reprinted with permission from Aphasia Institute.

APPENDIX 2

LANGUAGE-PROCESSING MODEL

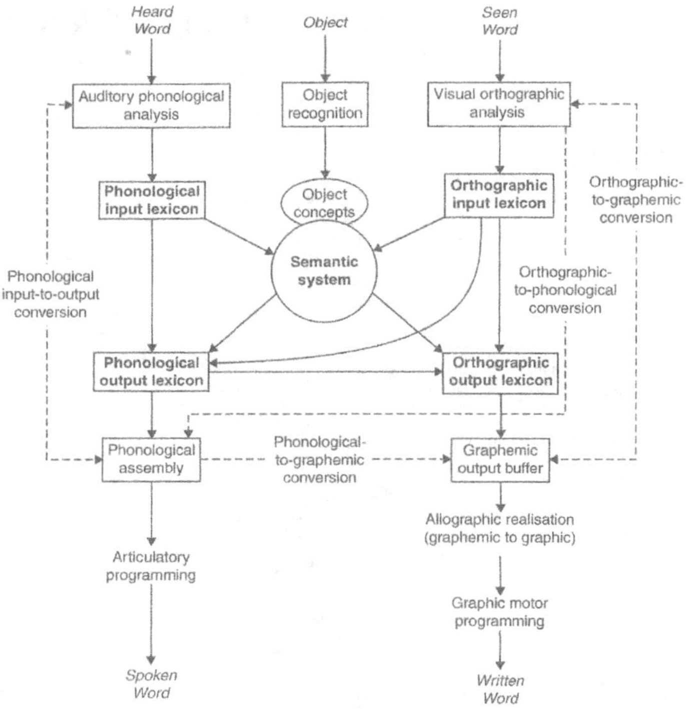

Figure 2.1 Language-Processing Model for single words, based on Patterson and Shewell's (1987) Logogen Model.

Source: Max Coltheart, Giuseppe Sartori and Remo Job (1987) *Cognitive Neuropsychology of Language*, Psychology Press. Reproduced by permission of Taylor & Francis Group.

APPENDIX 3

THE TOP TEN: BEST PRACTICE RECOMMENDATIONS FOR APHASIA (APHASIA UNITED "TOP 10")[1]

International Best Practice Recommendations for Aphasia

PREAMBLE

Aphasia is an acquired communication disability resulting from damage to the language areas of the brain, most often due to stroke, although other aetiologies such as brain trauma or tumour can also cause aphasia. Aphasia is characterised by impairments in language modalities including speaking, understanding, reading and writing. Because of the pervasive importance of communication in daily life, aphasia typically has a negative impact on social relationships, participation and well-being. People with aphasia have preserved pre-onset intelligence, but intelligence can be masked by difficulty communicating. It should never be assumed that a person with aphasia is mentally incompetent. People with aphasia are typically able to make decisions and participate in activities if information or activities are made communicatively accessible.

People with aphasia have the right to be treated with dignity and respect and to participate in the same level of healthcare as non-aphasic individuals (including obtaining information and participating in personally relevant decision making). People with aphasia and their family members have the right to relevant services designed for the individual to enhance communication and participation in life activities of choice. Healthcare services for people with aphasia should be person-centred and collaborative.

Following are "best practice recommendations" for healthcare or community services involving people with aphasia. These have been compiled from a variety of sources around the world. Sources are cited along with the level of recommendation/evidence cited in the source. Sources have not been directly quoted; rather, themes across cited sources have been worded to be representative. For more details on the levels of evidence please refer to the original source documents. It should be noted that most recommendations draw from general stroke guidelines, rather than other aetiologies or aphasia-specific guidelines.

TOP TEN BEST PRACTICE RECOMMENDATIONS FOR APHASIA

1. All patients with brain damage or progressive brain disease should be screened for communication deficits.[1,2,3,5,7,8,9] (Level C)
2. People with suspected communication deficits should be assessed by a qualified professional (determined by country); assessment should extend beyond the use of screening measures to determine the nature, severity and personal consequences of the suspected communication deficit.[1,2,3,4,5,6,8,9] (Levels B, C)
3. People with aphasia should receive information regarding aphasia, aetiologies of aphasia (e.g. stroke) and options for treatment.[1,5,6,7,8,9] (Levels A–C) This applies throughout all stages of healthcare from acute to chronic stages.
4. No one with aphasia should be discharged from services without some means of communicating his or her needs and wishes (e.g. using augmentative and alternative communication (AAC), supports, trained partners) or a documented plan for how and when this will be achieved. (Level: Good Practice Point)

5. People with aphasia should be offered intensive and individualised aphasia therapy designed to have a meaningful impact on communication and life.[1,2,3,4,5,6,7,8,9] (Level A-GPP depending on approach, intensity and timing). This intervention should be designed and delivered under the supervision of a qualified professional
   a. Intervention might consist of impairment-oriented therapy, compensatory training, conversation therapy, functional/participation-oriented therapy, environmental intervention and/or training in communication supports or augmentative and alternative communication (AAC.
   b. Modes of delivery might include individual therapy, group therapy, telerehabilitation and/or computer assisted treatment.
   c. Individuals with aphasia due to stable (e.g. stroke) as well as progressive forms of brain damage benefit from intervention.
   d. Individuals with aphasia due to stroke and other static forms of brain damage can benefit from intervention in both acute and chronic recovery phases.
6. Communication partner training should be provided to improve communication of the person with aphasia.[1,2,3,5,8] (Levels A, B)
7. Families or caregivers of people with aphasia should be included in the rehabilitation process.[1,2,3,4,5,7,8,9] (Levels A–C)
   a. Families and caregivers should receive education and support regarding the causes and consequences of aphasia. (Level A)
   b. Families and caregivers should learn to communicate with the person with aphasia. (Level B)
8. Services for people with aphasia should be culturally appropriate and personally relevant.[1,2,5,8] (Level: Good Practice Point)
9. All health and social care providers working with people with aphasia across the continuum of care (i.e. acute

care to end-of-life) should be educated about aphasia and trained to support communication in aphasia.[2,3] (Level C)
10. Information intended for use by people with aphasia should be available in aphasia friendly /communicatively accessible formats.[1,3,5,7,8] (Level C)

LEVELS OF RECOMMENDATION /EVIDENCE

Level A: Body of research evidence can be trusted to guide practice

Level B: Body of research evidence can be trusted to guide practice in most situations

Level C: Body of research evidence provides some support for recommendation

Level D: Body of research evidence is weak

Good Practice Point: Recommendation is based on expert opinion or consensus

PRIMARY SOURCES

1. Intercollegiate Stroke Working Party. (2012). *National Clinical Guideline for Stroke*, 4th edition. London: Royal College of Physicians.
2. Lindsay, M. P., Gubitz, G., Bayley, M., Hill, M. D., Davies-Schinkel, C., Singh, S., and Phillips, S. *Canadian Best Practice Recommendations for Stroke Care* (Update 2013). On behalf of the Canadian Stroke Strategy Best Practices and Standards Writing Group. Ottawa, Ontario Canada: Canadian Stroke Network.
3. Miller, E., Murray, L., Richards, L., Zorowitz, R., Bakas, T., Clark, P. Billinger, S. (2010). Comprehensive overview of nursing and interdisciplinary rehabilitation care of the stroke patient: a scientific statement from the American Heart Association. *Stroke*, 41: 2402–2448.
4. National Health and Medical Research Council Clinical Centre for Research Excellence in Aphasia Rehabilitation (CCRE) (2014). *Australian Aphasia Rehabilitation Pathway.*
5. National Stroke Foundation Australia (2010) *Clinical Guidelines for Stroke Prevention and Management.* Melbourne Australia.

http://strokefoundation.com.au/site/media/clinical_guidelines_stroke_managment_2010_interactive.pdf
6. Royal College of Speech & Language Therapists (2005). *RCSLT Clinical Guidelines*. London: RCSLT.
7. Scottish Intercollegiate Guidelines Network. (2010). *Management of Patients with Stroke: Rehabilitation, Prevention and Management of Complications, and Discharge Planning: A National Clinical Guideline*. Edinburgh, Scotland.
8. Stroke Foundation of New Zealand and New Zealand Guidelines Group. (2010). *Clinical Guidelines for Stroke Management 2010*. Wellington: Stroke Foundation of New Zealand.
9. US Veteran's Administration/Department of Defense. (2010). *Management of Stroke: VA/DoD Clinical Practice Guideline*. www.healthquality.va.gov/guidelines/Rehab/stroke/online

NOTE

1 Nina Simmons-Mackie, Linda Worrall, Laura L. Murray, Pam Enderby, Miranda L. Rose, Eun Jin Paek & Anu Klippi on behalf of the Aphasia United Best Practices Working Group and Advisory Committee (2017) The top ten: best practice recommendations. for aphasia, *Aphasiology*, 31:2, 131–151, doi: 10.1080/02687038.2016.1180662   https://doi.org/10.1080/02687038.2016.1180662

APPENDIX 4

SOME ASSESSMENTS

RATING SCALES

The **Aphasia Impact Questionnaire** is a formal rating scale within the CAT (Swinburn 2023) that asks the person with aphasia to give a subjective rating of the impact of the language difficulties identified in the Language Battery part of the CAT.

The **Aphasia Severity Rating (ASR)** is a single observational rating that was designed to provide an index of the severity of the aphasia language impairment. (Simmons-Mackie 2018). https://aphasia-institute.s3.amazonaws.com/uploads/2021/03/ASR-Rating-Scale.pdf

The **Assessment for Living with Aphasia (ALA)** is a self-rating measure of quality of life looking at someone's ability to perform various activities of daily living. It can be used to identify a person's communicative needs in everyday contexts (Simmons-Mackie 2014).

The **Communication Confidence Rating Scale for Aphasia (CCRSA)** (Babbitt et al., 2011) is a ten-item, self-rating scale looking at confidence in communicating.

The **Communicative Effectiveness Index (CETI)** (Lomas 1989) asks someone who knows the person with aphasia well to report on how effective their communication is in everyday life using a visual analogue scale.

The **Visual Analogue Self Esteem Scale (VASES)** (Brumfitt 1999b) is comprised of ten items and provides a reliable and valid measure of self-esteem.

Self-rating scales can rate someone's perception of different language skills, confidence, intelligibility, etc. They can provide useful baselines for comparison and reassessment during and after therapy.

Note that while these can form part of your picture of a client's aphasia, self-reports can be unreliable.

SCREENING TESTS

The Aphasia Screening Test (Whurr 1996).

The Frenchay Aphasia Screening Test (FAST) (Enderby, Wood & Wade (1987).

The Mississippi Aphasia Screening Test (MAST) (Nakase-Thompson 2004) has nine subtests and takes approximately 15 minutes to administer.

The Multimodal Communication Screening Test for Aphasia (MCST-A) (Garrett & Lasker 2005) forms part of the **AAC Assessment Battery for Aphasia (AAC-ABA)** for people with severe aphasia which aims to assess their ability to communicate using pictorial symbols and whether they can use them independently.

The Quick Aphasia Battery (QAB) (Wilson et al. 2018) has eight subtests and offers an assessment of language function at the bedside that takes about a quarter of an hour.

INTERVIEWS

O'Halloran, R., Worrall, L., Toffolo, D., Code, C., & Hickson, L. (2004). *Inpatient Functional Communication Interview: Manual.* Speech Mark.

INFORMAL ASSESSMENTS

The Life Interests and Values cards or the folder of Pictographic Resources from the Aphasia Institute (https://www.aphasia.ca)

could be used to guide a client through a discussion about their communication needs.

COGNITIVE FUNCTIONS

The Attention Network Test (ANT) (LaCroix 2021).

The CLQT (Cognitive Linguistic Quick Test) takes 15–30 minutes to administer and assesses attention, memory, executive functions, language and visuospatial skills.

The CoBaGA (Cognitive Test Battery for Global Aphasia) (Marinelli 2017) is a battery of nonverbal tests that assesses a wide range of cognitive functions (including attention, executive functions, memory, visual-auditory recognition and visual-spatial abilities).

The Cognitive Screen section of the CAT (Swinburn 2023) looks at some cognitive functions: visual neglect, access to semantic memory, nonverbal recognition memory and executive function (contrasting word fluency and picture naming) and includes a screen of ideomotor and ideational apraxia (gesture object use) and dyscalculia (arithmetic).

The Conversation Analysis Profile for People with Cognitive Impairment (CAPCI) (Perkins 1997)

The Measure of Cognitive Linguistic Abilities (MCLA) (Ellmo 1995).

The Test of Everyday Attention (TEA) (Robertson 1994)

GESTURE

The City Gesture Checklist (Caute, Dipper & Roper 2021) can be used to assess the types of gesture that people with aphasia produce. It describes itself as a 'quick and dirty' tool to analyse and record the types of gesture produced by people with aphasia. Preliminary findings suggest that clinicians can use it with a reasonable degree of reliability by following the checklist's written instructions.

A new bedside test of gestures in stroke: the **apraxia screen of TULIA** (AST) (Vanbellingen et al. 2010) is a reliable and valid bedside test for patients with stroke, allowing a straightforward assessment of apraxia within a few minutes.

FORMAL ASSESSMENTS OF LANGUAGE COMPREHENSION AND PRODUCTION

ABI

Cicerone, K. D., Smith, L. C., Ellmo, W., Mangel, H. R., Nelpartnern, P., Chase, R. F., & Kalmar, K. (1996). Neuropsychological rehabilitation of mild traumatic brain injury, *Brain Injury*, 10(4): 277–286. doi: 10.1080/026990596124458

Flanagan, S., McDonald, S., & Rollins, J. (2002). *The Awareness of Social Inference Test (TASIT)*. Pearson Assessment/PsychCorp.

Steel, J., Coluccio, I., Elbourn, E., & Spencer, E. (2023) How do speech-language pathologists assess and treat spoken discourse after TBI? A survey of clinical practice. *International Journal of Language & Communication Disorders*, 59(2): 591–607. doi: 10.1111/1460-6984.12784

Turner-Stokes, L., Kalmus, M., Hirani, D., & Clegg, F. (2005). The Depression Intensity Scale Circles (DISCS): a first evaluation of a simple assessment tool for depression in the context of brain injury. *Journal of Neurology, Neurosurgery and Psychiatry*, 76(9): 1273–1278. doi: 10.1136/jnnp.2004.050096

ASSESSING CONVERSATIONS

See conversation group wheel developed at the Wolfson (James, 2011).

James, K. (2011). *The Strands of Speech and Language Therapy: Weaving Plan for Neurorehabilitation*, p. 12, fig. 4 MPC/MSC (Measure of Level of Participation in Conversation/Measure of Skill in Supported Conversation).

Some assessments ask people to record conversations, e.g. Conversation Analysis Profile for People with Aphasia (CAPPA) (Whitworth, Perkins & Lesser 1997).

ASSESSING DISCOURSE

The Scenario Test (Hilari 2020) measures how a person with aphasia conveys everyday messages, verbally and/or non-verbally, in an interactive setting. There are six everyday scenarios and the person with aphasia adopts the role of a character who is faced with a communicative task.

CIU Analysis (Discourse Measures: Correct Information Unit Analysis) (Nicholas & Brookshire 1993).

This page provides information about approaches to discourse analysis: https://aphasia.talkbank.org/discourse

ASSESSMENT OF EMOTIONAL WELL-BEING/MOOD STATE

The SAQOL-39 (Hilari et al. 2003) includes questions about confidence and how much someone goes out and sees friends.

When verbal communication is limited, use non-verbal rating tools, e.g. the Visual Analogue Self-Esteem Scale (VASES) (Brumfitt 1999), a short and easy to administer measure of self-esteem. It also allows for the reading and/or writing difficulties someone with aphasia may have.

BILINGUAL CLIENTS

Some standardised assessments are translated into other languages, e.g. BDAE, Boston Naming Test, CADL,CAT, PALPA, WAB. The Bilingual Aphasia Test (BAT, Paradis 2011) can be used by non-SLT native speakers of the target language. Versions are available for free download.

Paradis, M. (2011). Principles underlying the Bilingual Aphasia Test (BAT) and its uses. *Clinical Linguistics & Phonetics*, 25(6–7): 427–443. doi: 10.3109/02699206.2011.560326. See www.mcgill.ca/linguistics/research/bat

Paradis, M., & Libben, G. (1987). *The Assessment of Bilingual Aphasia*. Lawrence Erlbaum.

Boston Diagnostic Aphasia Examination, 3rd ed. (Goodglass 2001).

The **CAT** (Comprehensive Aphasia Test) (Swinburn 2023) and **PALPA** (Psycholinguistic Assessments of Language Processing in Aphasia) (Kay 1992) follow a cognitive neuropsychological approach to understanding aphasia, building on models of language processing to design assessment tasks that identify the underlying language impairments.

The CAT is an aphasia battery or collection of assessments that begins to identify the underlying language impairments, suggests further assessments using PALPA and other batteries, suggests the impact of the aphasia on the client and creates a profile of strengths and weaknesses that can guide therapy. It also predicts and follows changes in severity over time. It has 34 subtests, including a cognitive screen, a language battery and an aphasia impact questionnaire (described under Rating scales, above). The cognitive screen looks at some deficits that your client may well have alongside the aphasia which can affect their ability to respond to therapy (e.g. visual processing, semantic and episodic memory). The language battery assesses: (1) language comprehension, (2) repetition, (3) spoken language production, (4) reading aloud and (5) writing. It is usually completed over two assessment sessions. You can compare the level of difficulty across the subtests and look at the client's communication strengths and weaknesses. The CAT tests also look at the effects of critical variables to further inform your understanding of the language impairments.

The PALPA is an assessment battery that provides a more in-depth examination of different areas of language. You can use the results from the CAT assessment to suggest which areas of language it would be useful to know more about to design therapy, and you can look to the PALPA to provide more relevant information. PALPA is a resource, not an assessment battery to administer in its entirety. There are 60 sub-tests, divided into four parts: (1) auditory processing, (2) reading and spelling, (3) picture and word semantics and (4) sentence comprehension. Like the CAT, PALPA tests look at the effects of critical variables and provide more items per sub-test to give more information about the underlying language impairments.

WAB (Western Aphasia Battery) (Kertesz 2007). This battery classifies the type and severity of aphasia and provides a clinically valid baseline for diagnosis, prognosis and research. Assesses linguistic skills: content, fluency, auditory comprehension, repetition, naming, reading, and writing. It assesses non-linguistic skills: drawing, calculation, block design and praxis. There are 8 subtests (32 short tasks). The full battery takes 30-45 minutes to administer, with a further 45-60 minutes for the reading, writing, praxis, and construction sections. The bedside version takes 15 minutes.

COGNITIVE ASSESSMENTS

Edmonds, L.A. (2014). Tutorial for Verb Network Strengthening Treatment (VNeST): detailed description of the treatment protocol with corresponding theoretical rationale. *Perspectives on Neurophysiology and Neurogenic Speech and Language Disorders*, 24(3): 78–88.

Edmonds, L. A.. (2016). A review of verb network strengthening treatment: theory, methods, results, and clinical implications. *Topics in Language Disorders* 36(2): 123–135. doi: 10.1097/TLD.0000000000000088

Ellmo, W., & Graser, J. (1995). *Measure of Cognitive Linguistic Abilities (MCLA)*. Speech Bin.

Enderby, P.M., Wood, V.A., Wade, D.T., & Hewer, R.L. (1987). The Frenchay Aphasia Screening Test: a short, simple test for aphasia appropriate for non-specialists. *International Rehabilitation Medicine*, 8(4):166–170. doi: 10.3109/03790798709166209

Helm-Estabrooks, N. (2001). *Cognitive Linguistic Quick Test: CLQT*. Psychological Corporation.

FUNCTIONAL COMMUNICATION

Communication Activities of Daily Living (CADL-3) (Holland, Frattali & Fromm 2018) examines the basic communication skills needed for daily living such as social interactions and non-verbal communication. There are 50 questions divided into categories such as reading, writing or using numbers, social interactions and divergent communication.

Simmons-Mackie, N., & Kagan, A. (2022). *Measure of Supported Conversation & Behaviour Change (MSCBC)*. Aphasia Institute. https://www.aphasia.ca/VF_MSCBC

For observational measures for rating support and participation see Kagan et al. (2004). www.aphasia.ca/health-care-providers/resources-and-tools/rating-scales/#ASR

IMPAIRMENT-BASED TOOLS

BDAE-3 (Goodglass 2001) is a comprehensive assessment battery that diagnoses someone's aphasia within the classification system. It measures performance over a wide range of tasks, to establish initial levels and detect change over time and assesses the strengths and impairments in five language-related sections: (1) conversational and expository speech, (2) auditory comprehension, (3) oral expression, (4) understanding written language and (5) writing. Each section contains a variety of sub-tests. There is a standard and shortened version. The assessment of narrative speech includes the description of a line drawing (the 'cookie theft"'card).

OTHER ASSESSMENTS THAT LOOK AT AREAS OF LANGUAGE PERFORMANCE

Bishop, D. (2003). Test for Reception of Grammar, 2nd ed. Pearson.

Bstinaanse, R., Edwards, S., & Reispens, J. (2002). Verb and Sentence Test. Thames Valley Test Company.

DeRenzi, E., Vignolo, L. A. (1962). The Token Test — a sensitive test to detect receptive disturbances in aphasias. *Brain*, 85: 556–678.

Howard, D., & Patterson, K. (1992). *The Pyramids and Palm Trees Test. A Test of Semantic Access from Words and Pictures.* Thames Valley Company.

Kaplan, E., Goodglass, H., & Weintraub, S. (2000). *Boston Naming Test.* Lippincott Williams & Wilkins Publishers UK.

LaPointe, L.L., & Horner, J. (1998). *Reading Comprehension Battery for Aphasia*, 2nd ed. (RCBA-2), *Examiners Manual*. Pro-Ed.

McKenna & Warrington (1983). *Graded Naming Test*

The Philadelphia Naming Battery (Roach et al. 1996) is available for free and downloadable from the Moss Rehabilitation website (https://mrri.org/philadelphia-naming-test).

OTHER AREAS

Bryan, K.L. (1988), Assessment of language disorders after right hemisphere damage. *International Journal of Language & Communication Disorders*, 23: 111–125. https://doi.org/10.3109/13682828809019881

Bryan, K. (1994). *Right Hemisphere Language Battery*, 2nd ed. Whurr Publishers.

Dabul, B. (2000). *Apraxia Battery for Adults*, 2nd ed. Pro-Ed Inc.

Enderby, P., & Palmer, R. (1983). *The Frenchay Dysarthria Assessment*. Pro-Ed.

Enderby, P., & Palmer, R. (2008). *Frenchay Dysarthria Assessment*, 2nd ed. Pro-Ed Inc.

Jacobson, B. H., Johnson, A., Grywalski, C., Silbergleit, A., Jacobson, G., Benninger, M.S., & Newman, C.W. (1997). The Voice Handicap Index (VHI): development and validation. *American Journal of Speech-Language Pathology*, 6(3): 66–70.

Kopelman, M., Wilson, B.A., & Baddeley, A.D. (1989). The autobiographical memory interview: a new assessment of autobiographical and personal semantic memory in amnesic patients. *Journal of Clinical and Experimental Neuropsychology*, 11(5): 724–744. doi: 10.1080/01688638908400928..

Robertson, S. J. (1987). *Communication Skills*. Builders Inc.

Vanbellingen, T., Kersten, B., Van Hemelrijk, B., Van de Winckel, A., Bertschi, M., Müri, R., De Weerdt, W., & Bohlhalter, S. (2010). Comprehensive assessment of gesture production: a new test of upper limb apraxia (TULIA). *European Journal of Neurology*, 17(1): 59–66. doi: 10.1111/j.1468-1331.2009.02741 (The AST Apraxia Screen of TULIA – Test for Upper-Limb Apraxia (TULIA) is a short and validated diagnostic test of people after a stroke that diagnoses apraxia.)

Yorkston, K. M., & Beukelman, D., (1981). *Assessment of Intelligibility of Dysarthric Speech*. Pro-Ed.

Arizona Battery for Communication Disorders of Dementia (ABCD), *Western Aphasia Battery – Revised (WAB-R) (*Kertesz 2007), Sever Impairment Battery (SIB), observations.

Functional Linguistic Communication Inventory (FLCI-2) (Bayles & Tomoeda 2010) is a standardized test battery that assesses the functional language of patients with moderate to severe dementia. The inventory measures communication skills such as greeting and naming, comprehension of signs/object-to-picture matching, following commands, and conversation.

QUALITY OF LIFE

Adult Carers Quality of Life questionnaire (Joseph et al., 2012).

American Speech-Language-Hearing Association (ASHA) Quality of Communication Life Quality of Communication Life Scale (ASHA QCL) (Frattali et al. 2017).

The Stroke and Aphasia Quality of Life Scale-39 (SAQOL) (Hilari 2001) is a health related, quality of life, patient-reported outcome measure.

REFERENCES

Babbitt, E. M., Heinemann, A. W., Semik, P., & Cherney, L. R. (2011). *Communication Confidence Rating Scale for Aphasia (CCRSA).*

Bayles, K. & Tomoeda, C.K. (2010). *Functional Linguistic Communication Inventory (FLCI-2)*, Slosson Inc.

Babbitt, E. M., Cherney, L. R. (2010). Communication confidence in persons with aphasia. *Top Stroke Rehabilitation*, 17(3): 214-223. doi: 10.1310/tsr1703-214

https://aphasiology.pitt.edu/2167/1/viewpaper.pdf

Caute, A., Dipper, L., & Roper, A. (2021), The City Gesture Checklist: the development of a novel gesture assessment. *International Journal of Language & Communication Disorders*, 56: 20–35. https://doi.org/10.1111/1460-6984.12579

Ellmo, W., & Graser, J. (1995). *Measure of Cognitive Linguistic Abilities (MCLA)*. Speech Bin.

Frattali, C. M., Thompson, C. K., Holland, A. L., Wohl, C. B., Wenck, C. J., Slater, S. C., & Paul, D. (2017). *American Speech-Language-Hearing Association Functional Assessment of Communication Skills for Adults.* American Speech-Language-Hearing Association.

Garrett, K., & Lasker, J., (2005). *The Multimodal Communication Screening Task for Persons with Aphasia (MCST) – A.* Revised ed. University of Nebraska-Lincoln Department of Special Education & Communication Disorders https://aac.unl.edu/materials/aphasia-assessment-materials

Hilari, K., Byng, S., Lamping, D. L., & Smith, S. C. (2003). Stroke and Aphasia Quality of Life Scale-39 (SAQOL-39): evaluation of acceptability, reliability, and validity. *Stroke*, 34(8): 1944–1950. https:// doi.org/10.1161/01.STR.0000081987.46660.ED 01.STR.0000081987.46660.ED [pii]

Hilari, K., & Dipper, L. (2020). *The Scenario Test*. J&R Press.

Holland, A. L., Frattali, C., & Fromm, D. (2018). *Communication Activities of Daily Living*, 3rd ed. Pro-Ed Press.

Joseph, S., Becker, S., Elwick, H., & Silburn, R. (2012). Adult Carers Quality of Life Questionnaire (AC-QoL): development of an evidence-based tool. *Mental Health Review Journal*, 17: 57–69.

Kagan, A., Winckel, J., Black, S., Duchan, J., Simmons-Mackie, N., & Square, P. (2004). A set of observational measures for rating support and participation in conversation between adults with aphasia and their conversation partners. *Topics in Stroke Rehabilitation*, 11(1): 67–83. https://doi.org/10.1310/CL3V-A94A-DE5C-CVBE

Kay, J., Lesser, R., & Coltheart, M. (1992) *Psycholinguistic Assessments of Language Processing in Aphasia (PALPA)*. Lawrence Erlbaum Associates.

Kertesz, A. (2007). *Western Aphasia Battery—Revised (WAB-R)*. Pearson.

LaCroix, A. N., Tully, M., & Rogalsky, C. (2021). Assessment of alerting, orienting, and executive control in persons with aphasia using the Attention Network Test. *Aphasiology*, 35(10): 1318–1333. doi: 10.1080/02687038.2020.1795077

Lomas, J., Pickard, L., Bester, S., Zoghaib, C. (1989) The Communication Effectiveness Index: Development and psychometric evaluation of a functional communication measure for adult aphasia. *Journal of Speech and Hearing Disorders*, 54(1), 113–124.

Marinelli, C. V., Spaccavento, S., Craca, A., Marangolo, P., & Angelelli, P. (2017). Different cognitive profiles of patients with severe aphasia. *Behavioural Neurology*, 2017(1): 3875954. doi: 10.1155/2017/3875954

Nakase-Thompson, R. (2004). *The Mississippi Aphasia Screening Test*. The Center for Outcome Measurement in Brain Injury. https://www.tbims.org/mast/index.html

Perkins, L., Whitworth, A., & Lesser, R. (1997). *Conversation Analysis Profile for People with Cognitive Impairment (CAPCI)*. Whurr Publishers.

Roach, A., Schwartz, M. F., Martin, N., Grewal, R. S., & Brecher, A. (1996). *The Philadelphia Naming Test: Scoring and Rationale*.

APA PsychNet Direct https://psycnet.apa.org/doiLanding?doi=10.1037%2Ft56477-000

Robertson, I. H., Ward, T., Ridgeway, V., & Nimmo-Smith, I. (1994). *The Test of Everyday Attention (TEA)*. Psychological Corporation.

Simmons-Mackie, N., Kagan, A., Victor, J. C., Carling-Rowland, A., Mok, A., Hoch, J. S., Huijbregts, M., & Streiner, D. L. (2014). The assessment for living with aphasia: reliability and construct validity. *International Journal Speech-Lang Pathology*, 16(1): 82–94. doi: 10.3109/17549507.2013.831484

Simmons-Mackie, N., Kagan, A., & Shumway, E. (2018). *Aphasia Severity Rating*. Aphasia Institute, Canada.

Swinburn, K., Porter, G., & Howard, D. (2023). *The Comprehensive Aphasia Test (CAT)*, 2nd ed. Routledge.

Vanbellingen, T., Kersten, B., Van Hemelrijk, B., Van de Winckel, A., Bertschi, M., Müri, R., De Weerdt, W., & Bohlhalter, S. (2010). Comprehensive assessment of gesture production: a new test of upper limb apraxia (TULIA). *European Journal of Neurology*, 17(1): 59–66.

Whitworth, A., Perkins, L., & Lesser, R. (1997) *Conversation Analysis Profile for People with Aphasia (CAPPA)*. Whurr Publishers.

Whurr, R. (1996). *Aphasia Screening Test*. Whurr Publishers.

Wilson, S. M., Eriksson, D. K., Schneck, S. M., Lucanie J. M. (2018). A quick aphasia battery for efficient, reliable, and multidimensional assessment of language function. *PLoS One* 13(2): e0192773.

FURTHER READING

Armstrong, E., Bryant, L., Ferguson, A., & Simmons-Mackie, N. (2012). Approaches to assessment and treatment of everyday talk in aphasia. In I. Papathanasiou & P. Coppens (Eds.), *Aphasia and Related Neurogenic Communication Disorders*, 2nd ed. (pp. 269–285). Jones & Barlett Learning.

Australian Aphasia Rehabilitation Pathway: Aphasia Assessment and the ICF: https://www.aphasiapathway.com.au/?name=ICF-and-aphasia-assessments

Babbitt, E. M., Heinemann, A. W., Semik, P., & Cherney, L. R. (2011). *Communication Confidence Rating Scale for Aphasia*. CCRSA

Baker, C., Ryan, B., & El-Helou, R. (2022). Mood screening tools for people with aphasia. *Journal of Clinical Practice in*

Speech-Language Pathology, 24(3): 148. https://doi.org/10.1080/22087168.2022.12370376

Bastiaanse, R., Edwards, S., & Rispens, J. (2002). *Verb and Sentence Test (VAST)*. Thames Valley Test Company.

Bayles, K., & Tomoeda, C. K. (2010). *Functional Linguistic Communication Inventory (FLCI-2),*. Pro-Ed.

Brumfitt, S. M., & Sheeran, P. (1999a). The development and validation of the Visual Analogue Self-Esteem Scale (VASES). *British Journal of Clinical Psychology*, 38(4): 387–400. doi: 10.1348/014466599162980

Brumfitt, S. & Sheeran, P. (1999b). *Visual Analogue Self Esteem Scale (VASES)*. Speechmark Publishing.

Caute, A., Dipper, L., & Roper, A. (2021). The City Gesture Checklist: the development of a novel gesture assessment. *International Journal of Language & Communication Disorders* 56(1); 20–35.

Ellmo, W., & Graser, J. (1995). *Measure of Cognitive Linguistic Abilities (MCLA)*. Speech Bin.

Enderby, P., Wood, V., & Wade, D. (1987). *Frenchay Aphasia Screening Test*. NFER-Nelson.

Franklin, S., Turner, J., Ellis, A .(1992). *The ADA Comprehension Battery*. Human Neuropyschology Laboratory, University of York. Distribution through Action for Dysphasic Adults, 1 Royal St., London SE1.

Garrett, K., & Lasker, J., (2005). *The Multimodal Communication Screening Task for Persons with Aphasia (MCST) – A*. Revised ed. https://aac.unl.edu/materials/aphasia-assessment-materials

Goodglass, H., Kaplan, E., & Barresi, B. (2001). *Boston Diagnostic Aphasia Examination (BDAE)*, 3rd ed. Pearpartner.

Helm-Estabrooks, N. (2001). *Cognitive Linguistic Quick Test*. The Psychological Corporation.

Hilari, K., & Byng, S. (2001). Measuring quality of life in people with aphasia: the Stroke Specific Quality of Life Scale. *International Journal of Language Communication Disorders*, 36(Suppl.): 86–91.

Hilari, K., Byng, S., Lamping, D. L., & Smith, S. C. (2003). The Stroke and Aphasia Quality of Life Scale-39 (SAQOL-39): evaluation of acceptability, reliability and validity. *Stroke*, 34(8): 1944–1950.

Hilari, K. & Dipper, L. (2020). *The Scenario Tes.t* J&R Press.

Holland, A.L., Frattali, C., & Fromm, D. (2018). *Communication Activities of Daily Living*, 3rd ed. Pro-Ed Press.

Holland, A. (1980). *CADL: Communicative Abilities in Daily Living. A Test of Functional Communication for Aphasic Adults.* University Park Press.

Howard, D., Patterson, K. (1992). *The Pyramids and Palm Trees Test: A Test of Semantic Access from Words to Pictures.* Thames Valley Test Company.

Joseph, S., Becker, S., Elwick, H., & Silburn, R. (2012). Adult Carers Quality of Life Questionnaire (AC-QoL): development of an evidence-based tool. *Mental Health Review Journal,* 17: 57–69.

Kagan, A., Simmons-Mackie, N., & Shumway, E. (2018). *Revised Rating Anchors and Scoring Procedures for Measure of Skill and Measure of Participation in Conversation between Adults with Aphasia and Their Conversation Partners.* Aphasia Institute. https://www.aphasia.ca/VF_MSCMPC

Kagan, A., Winckel, J., Black, S., Duchan, J., Simmons-Mackie, N., & Square, P. (2004). A set of observational measures for rating support and participation in conversation between adults with aphasia and their conversation partners. *Topics in Stroke Rehabilitation,* 11(1): 67–83. https://doi.org/10.1310/CL3V-A94A-DE5C-CVBE

Kertesz, A. (2007). *Western Aphasia Battery—Revised (WAB-R).* Pearson.

LaCroix, A. N., Tully, M., & Rogalsky, C. (2021). Assessment of alerting, orienting, and executive control in persons with aphasia using the Attention Network Test. *Aphasiology,* 35(10): 1318–1333. doi: 10.1080/02687038.2020.1795077

Laska, A., Bartfai, A., Hellblom, A., Murray, V., & Kahan, T., 2007, Clinical and prognostic properties of standardised and functional aphasia assessment. *Journal of Rehabilitation Medicine,* 39(5): 387–392.

Lesser, K. J., & Coltheart, M. (1992) *Psycholinguistic Assessments of Language Processing in Aphasia (PALPA).* Lawrence Erlbaum Associates.

Lomas, J., Pickard, L., Bester, S., & Zoghaib, C. (1989) The Communication Effectiveness Index: development and psychometric evaluation of a functional communication measure for adult aphasia. *Journal of Speech and Hearing Disorders,* 54(1), 113–124.

Measure of Cognitive Linguistic Abilities (MCLA), Ellmo W & Graser J (1995) Speech Bin, Vero Beach, FL.

Nakase-Thompson, R. (2004). *The Mississippi Aphasia Screening Test*. The Center for Outcome Measurement in Brain Injury. https://www.tbims.org/mast/index.html

Nicholas, L. E., & Brookshire, R. H. (1993). A system for quantifying the informativeness and efficiency of the connected speech of adults with aphasia. *Journal of Speech and Hearing Research*, 36(2): 338–350. https://doi.org/10.1044/jshr.3602.338

Perkins, L., Whitworth, A., & Lesser, R. (1997). *Conversation Analysis Profile for People with Cognitive Impairment (CAPCI)*. Whurr Publishers.

Roach, A., Schwartz, M. F., Martin, N., Grewal, R. S., & Brecher, A. (1996). The Philadelphia Naming Test: scoring and rationale. *Clinical Aphasiology*, 24: 121–133.

Robertson, I. H., Ward, T., Ridgeway, V., & Nimmo-Smith, I. (1994). *The Test of Everyday Attention (TEA)*. Psychological Corporation.

Simmons-Mackie, N., Kagan, A., Victor, J. C., Carling-Rowland, A., Mok, A., Hoch, J. S., Huijbregts, M., & Streiner, D. L. (2014). The assessment for living with aphasia: reliability and construct validity. *International Journal Speech-Lang Pathology*, 16(1): 82–94. doi: 10.3109/17549507.2013.831484

Simmons-Mackie, N., Kagan, A., & Shumway, E. (2018). *Aphasia Severity Rating*. Aphasia Institute, Canada.

Sutcliffe, L. M., & Lincoln, N. B. (1998). The assessment of depression in aphasic stroke patients: the development of the Stroke Aphasic Depression Questionnaire. *Clinical Rehabilitation*, 12(6): 506–513. https://doi.org/10.1191/026921598672167702

Swinburn, K., Porter, G., & Howard, D. (2023). *The Comprehensive Aphasia Test (CAT)*, 2nd ed. Routledge.

Vanbellingen, T., Kersten, B., Van Hemelrijk, B., Van de Winckel, A., Bertschi, M., Müri, R., De Weerdt, W., & Bohlhalter, S. (2010). Comprehensive assessment of gesture production: a new test of upper limb apraxia (TULIA). *European Journal of Neurology*, 17(1): 59–66.

Whitworth, A., Perkins, L., & Lesser, R. (1997). *Conversation Analysis Profile for People with Aphasia (CAPPA)*. Whurr Publishers.

Whurr, R. (1995). The assessment of aphasia: a review of aphasia assessments, batteries, evaluations and procedures 1886–1996. *International Journal of Language & Communication Disorders*, 30(1): 377–378. https://doi.org/10.1111/j.1460-6984.1995.tb01706.x

Wilson, S. M., Eriksson, D. K., Schneck, S. M., Lucanie J. M. (2018). A quick aphasia battery for efficient, reliable, and multidimensional assessment of language function. *PLoS One* 13(2): e0192773.

www.rcslt.info/how-to-formal-assessments provides e-learning, including video content, of the CAT and PALPA assessments being carried out.

APPENDIX 5

USEFUL RESOURCES, LINKS AND WEBSITES

SOME CLINICAL GUIDELINES

Aphasia therapy CEN – via RCSLT and on X @aphasia_CEN – a Clinical Excellence Network that provides study days and information for SLTs.

Australian Aphasia Rehabilitation Pathway (2014). *Best Practice Statements Comprehensive Supplement to the Australian Aphasia Rehabilitation Pathway.* http://www.aphasiapathway.com.au/fluxcontent/aarp/pdf/Aphasia-Rehabilitation-Best-Practice-Statements-15042015-comprehensive-BMJ-Suppl-file-b.pdf

Headway – the brain injury association https://www.headway.org.uk/media/3320/bsrm-rehabilitation-following-acquired-brain-injury.pdf

Intercollegiate Stroke Working Party (2023). *National Clinical Guideline for Stroke for the UK and Ireland.* London: Intercollegiate Stroke Working Party (2023) www.strokeguideline.org.

National Institute for Health and Care Excellence (NICE). (2023, 18 October) Guideline [NG236] Published: 18 October 2023 Stroke *Rehabilita*tion in *Adults Clinical Guideline,* NG236. https://www.nice.org.uk/guidance/ng236

National Institute for Health and Care Research (NIHR) https://evidence.nihr.ac.uk/alert/therapy-for-language

-problems-after-a-stroke-is-most-effective-when-given-early-and-intensively/

Royal College of Speech and Language Therapists: clinical guidance https://www.rcslt.org/members/clinical-guidance/stroke/stroke-guidance/#section-11

Royal College of Speech and Language Therapists: clinical guidance https://www.rcslt.org/wp-content/uploads/media/Project/RCSLT/aphasia-resource-updated-feb-2014.pdf

See Appendix 3 for Aphasia United Aphasia United – School of Health and Rehabilitation Sciences – University of Queensland (uq.edu.au) list of the Top 10 best practice recommendations for aphasia using clinical guidelines drawn from general stroke guidelines, e.g. Intercollegiate Stroke Working Party. (2012). Aphasia-recommendations-English.pdf (uq.edu.au)

SOME APHASIA ORGANISATIONS

IN THE UK

- **Aphasia Alliance** is a coalition of key organisations from all over the UK that work in the field of aphasia. https://aphasiaaliiance.og/members
- **Aphasia Support** is a registered charity that works across Yorkshire helping people with aphasia work on communication goals which have been identified by themselves with the support of SLTs and their carers. https://aphasiasupport.org
- **Association for Speech & Language Therapists in Independent Practice (ASLTIP)** provides information and a contact point for members of the public searching for an independent speech and language therapist. It also provides members with access to a UK network of SLTs and ongoing professional support. www.helpwithtalking.com
- **Connect** provides a peer support network of people living with aphasia, with face-to-face groups in London and online groups for conversation and support. https://aphasiareconnect.org

- **Dyscover** is a charity providing long-term support and opportunities to people with aphasia and their families in Surrey and South London. It follows the LPAA approach and uses supported conversation across the service with its daily sessions led by speech and language therapists and designed to help people to adjust to living with aphasia. https://www.dyscover.org.uk
- **North East Trust for Aphasia (NETA)** is a charity supporting people in the north-east of England with aphasia and their families. It offers long-term support to people with aphasia through the NETA Aphasia Support Centre, and its various groups. NETA also aims to raise awareness of aphasia in the general public. https://www.neta.org.uk
- **Say Aphasia** helps people with aphasia adapt to their new way of life and regain independence and confidence. Groups meet in person in Abergavenny, Cardiff, Bournemouth, Chichester, Crawley, Burgess Hill, Darlington, Eastbourne, Exeter, Hove, Selsey, Skipton, Southampton, Winchester, Woodingdean and Worthing and online. https://www.sayaphasia.org
- **Speakeasy** is a specialist aphasia charity supporting people affected by aphasia in the north-west of England that provides groups. http://speakeasy-aphasia.org.uk
- Stroke Association provides information and support and Stroke Clubs. https://www.stroke.org.uk/what-is-aphasia
- **The Intensive Comprehensive Aphasia Programme @ Queen Square** is for adults who have aphasia caused by an acquired brain injury, usually stroke, brain tumours or head injury. https://www.ucl.ac.uk/icn/research/research-groups/neurotherapeutics/leff-lab/leff-lab-nhs-clinical-services/intensive
- **The Tavistock Aphasia Centre** at the University of Newcastle https://www.ncl.ac.uk/ecls/about-us/facilities/tavistock-aphasia-centre provides speech and language therapy for people with aphasia, training for its SLT students, engages in aphasia research and works with NETA.

- **The Tavistock Trust for Aphasia** is the only grant making trust in the United Kingdom to focus solely on aphasia. It aims to help improve the quality of life for those with aphasia, their families and carers. It website has a number of useful links including to the aphasia software finder. https://aphasiatavistocktrust.org

IN THE USA

- Aphasia Access www.aphasiaaccess.orgNational Aphasia Association (USA) https://aphasia.org
- ARC Aphasia Recovery Connection https://www.aphasiarecoveryconnection.net
- Stroke Onward https://strokeonward.org
- Triangle Aphasia Project https://www.aphasiaproject.org

IN CANADA

- Aphasia Friendly Canada https://aphasiafriendlycanada.ca
- The Aphasia Institute (incorporating the Pat Arato Aphasia Centre) in Toronto www.aphasia.ca

IN AUSTRALIA

- Australian Aphasia Association https://aphasia.org.au
- La Trobe University Centre for Research Excellence in Aphasia Recovery and Rehabilitation https://www.latrobe.edu.au/research/centres/health/aphasia
- Talkback Association for Aphasia https://aphasia.asn.au

IN INDIA

- Aphasia and Stroke Association of India https://www.aphasiastrokeindia.com

IN IRELAND

- Aphasia Ireland https://www.aphasiaireland.ie

INFORMATION AND THERAPY RESOURCES FOR CLINICIANS

ABI A programme for people with traumatic brain injury and their family, friends or carers have better conversations together: https://www.sydney.edu.au/medicine-health/our-research/research-centres/acquired-brain-injury-communication-lab/tbiconnect.html

AphasiaBank is an online database of discourse samples and assessment results from volunteers with aphasia. Its collections are available to members to use for research into aphasia. https://aphasia.talkbank.org

The training at the **Aphasia Institute** is based on Supported Conversation for Adults with Aphasia (SCA™) techniques developed at the Institute. You will learn how to work with clients to overcome the communication barriers aphasia creates, enable access to your services and help clients re-engage in everyday life. https://www.aphasia.ca/health-care-providers/education-training

Aphasia Institute free online e-learning: Supported Conversation for Adults with Aphasia (SCA™) (60 minutes)

See the Aphasia Institute website for resources, e.g. *Talking to Your Doctor, Talking about Transport*. The publications use supported conversation techniques to enable conversations about topics between people with aphasia and others in their lives, e.g. health professionals or someone at the bank. https://www.aphasia.ca

Aphasia Therapy Finder, a project of CATS (Collaboration of Aphasia Trialists), is a database of 25 evidence-based therapies for aphasia with descriptions of therapy, resources and summaries of the evidence for the therapy. It has step-by-step instructions, including videos, and links to therapy resources. www.aphasiatherapyfinder.com Dignam, J. K., Harvey, S., Monnelly, K., Dipper, L., Hoover, E., Kirmess, M., … Rose, M. L. (2023). Development of an evidence-based aphasia therapy implementation tool: an international survey of speech pathologists' access to and use of aphasia therapy resources.

Aphasiology, 38(6): 1051–1068. https://doi.org/10.1080/02687038.2023.2253994).

British Aphasiology Society (BAS) is a national interest group formed to foster the study of aphasia and promote development of a range of clinical services for people with aphasia. It is well worth joining the BAS for the opportunities it provides to continue learning about aphasia and aphasia therapy: monthly research summaries of recent peer-reviewed articles on aphasia, the annual BAS Research Update Meeting and the BAS International Conference and therapy masterclasses which provide a theoretical overview and practical guidance about aphasia therapy. There are support funds to attend BAS and non-BAS events, cash prizes for student work related to aphasia and research funding for small projects. Aphasia Therapy Masterclasses cover a specific aphasia intervention or approach, including discussion relating to a relevant evidence-based case-study, and discussion and a video of implementation and the opportunity for questions and answers. https://www.bas.org.uk

Communication and dementia University of Newcastle DemTalk toolkit for health and care professionals http://www.demtalk.org.uk/healthcareprofessionals

Life Participation Approach to Aphasia (LPAA) supply videos, including core values and techniques. https://www.aphasiaaccess.org/videos

SFA Therapy resource *The Epworth Aphasia Therapy Manual* contains single word treatment materials targeting the semantic system and output lexicons as well as videos demonstrating these resources being used.

speechBITE is an online database established to help speech and language therapists gain faster access to relevant research that can used in clinical decision-making. https://speechbite.com/about; www.speechbite.com

The Centre for Aphasia and Related Disorders at UNC School of Medicine, North Carolina is an education and research centre. This goal pool shares experience and knowledge of planning aphasia therapy. https://www.med.unc.edu/health-sciences/sphs/card/resources/aphasia-goals/goal-pool

The Centre for Language and Communication Science Research at City University, London carries out research into all aspects of speech, language and communication disorders, https://researchcentres.city.ac.uk/language-and-communication-science

The Collaboration of Aphasia Trialists (CATs) is an international network of multidisciplinary aphasia investigators in rehabilitation, social science, psychology and linguistics research from across more than 50 countries. https://www.aphasiatrials.org/https://www.aphasiatrials.org

The Communication Disability Network (2013). *Better Conversations: A Guide for Relatives of People with Communication Disability*. Connect.

See also Connect ideas series: *Caring and Coping, Having a Stroke, Being a Parent, How to Volunteer*.

Learn how to do conversation therapy with access to a complete therapy programme, interactive learning materials and advice from experienced clinicians. https://www.ucl.ac.uk/short-courses/search-courses/better-conversations-aphasia-e-learning-resource

Beeke, S., Sirman, N., Beckley, F., Maxim, J., Edwards, S., Swinburn, K., & Best, W. (2013). Better conversations with aphasia: An e-learning resource. https://extend.ucl.ac.uk

Boardmaker Picture Index. (1996). *The Picture Communication Symbols*. Mayer-Johnson Co.

Laird, L. (2008). Treating naming impairments in aphasia: Findings from a phonological components analysis treatment. *Aphasiology*, 22(9), 923–947.

Morris, J., Webster, J., Whitworth, A., & Howard, D. (2009). *Auditory Processing Resources*. University of Newcastle upon Tyne

Narrative and Discourse Intervention in Aphasia Team https://nadiiatherapy.com

Snodgrass, J. G., & Vanderwart, M. (1980). A standardized set of 260 pictures: norms for name agreement, image agreement, familiarity, and visual complexity. *Journal of Experimental Psychology: Human Learning and Memory*, 6i: 174–215.

Tactus Therapy https://tactustherapy.com/pca-phonological-components-analysis-aphasia

The Aphasia Therapy Finder https://aphasiatherapyfinder.com/dashboard

Training Communication Partners of People with Acquired Brain Injury (TANGO).. www.blogs.city.ac.uk/TANGO

University of Queensland Language Neuroscience Laboratory https://aphasialab.org/resources

Webster, J., Morris, J., Whitworth, A., & Howard, D. (2009). *Newcastle University Aphasia Therapy Resources*. University of Newcastle upon Tyne.

THERAPY RESOURCES FOR CLINICIANS AND CLIENTS

Adler Aphasia Center: https://www.youtube.com/watch?v=bAaPWwE_xUI

Aphasia Information Pack
https://aphasiareconnect.org/wp-content/uploads/2019/04/AphasiaInformationPack.pdf

Aphasia Therapy Online (free resource) www.aphasiatherapyonline.com

Stroke Association (UK) Scottish Acquired Brain Injury Network eLearning resource https://www.acquiredbraininjury-education.scot.nhs.uk/what-is-acquired-brain-injury

Stroke Foundation Australia sf1629_aphasia-booklet.pdf (strokefoundation.org.au) and
https://strokefoundation.org.au/media/c3qjm2zw/sf1629_aphasia-booklet.pdf

Stroke Onward https://strokeonward.org

APHASIA SOFTWARE

Aphasia Software Finder https://www.aphasiasoftwarefinder.org It provides software including:

- Aphasia Therapy Online http://www.aphasiatherapyonline.com
- Bitboard http://bitsboard.com
- CueSpeak https://cuespeak.com/clinicians
    - React2 https://www.react2.com
    - Sentence Shaper https://sentenceshaper.comStep-by-step V5 https://www.steps.uk
    - Speech Sounds on Cue https://mmsp.com.au/product/speech-sounds-on-cue-for-iphone-and-ipad
    - Tactus Therapy https://tactustherapy.com

AAC

American Speech-Language-Hearing Association: Augmentative and Alternative Communication (AAC) https://www.asha.org/Practice-Portal/Professional-Issues/Augmentative-and-Alternative-Communication

Speech Pathology Australia: Augmentative and Alternative Communication https://www.speechpathologyaustralia.org.au/Public/Public/Comm-swallow/Aug-alt-strategies/Augmentative-Alternative-Communication.aspx

APHASIA GROUPS ONLINE

Aphasia Access
Aphasia Awareness
Aphasia Communication group – Aphasia Centre of California
Aphasia NYC – People will Talk: Aphasia Group
Aphasia Re-connect (UK)
Aphasia Recovery Connection (ARC)
Aphasia Support (UK) https://aphasiasupport.org
Better Conversations with Aphasia
Drawing for People with Aphasia (London, UK)
Dyscover https://www.dyscover.org.uk

Korero Clubs & Groups (New Zealand) https://www.aphasia
.org.nz/aphasianz-services/support-meetings
National Aphasia Association (USA)
NETA – North East Trust for Aphasia
Say Aphasia (UK) https://www.sayaphasia.org/
Sing Aphasia
Triangle Aphasia Project Unlimited

GLOSSARY

ABI   acquired brain injury.
Acalculia   a disorder of number processing and/or calculation.
Agrammatism   difficulties with processing sentences, involving both comprehension and production of sentences. Agrammatic speech is non-fluent, made up mainly of content words with few verbs and little sentence structure.
Agraphia/dysgraphia   a disorder of writing or spelling.
Anomia   difficulties with word retrieval/word finding involving delays and failures. Most people with aphasia have some anomia.
Anoxia   is the complete loss of oxygen supply to the body's tissues, e.g. the brain. Partial loss of oxygen is known as hypoxia.
Argument structure   the argument in a sentence is built around the verb and the pattern of thematic roles that the verb takes.
Articulate, articulatory programming   the process of organising the neuromuscular system to produce phonemes in speech via, for example, e.g. the tongue or the lips.
Atrophy   brain atrophy is a loss of neurons and connections between neurons often with a decrease in brain volume. It may be focal or generalised. It may result from ABI, stroke or dementia.
Auditory phonological analysis   the process of identifying speech sounds via analysis of sounds heard. A deficit here can lead to word sound deafness.
Automatic speech   is often prompted by the clinician and completed 'automatically', e.g. serial speech such as days of the week or numbers. It can also involve rhymes, poems and song lyrics and well-known sayings.

Baselines are taken to measure changes and/or progress in language skills and communication abilities, in someone's well-being and life participation. They are taken before, during and after therapy. They contribute to decisions on the type of therapy and its impact.

Circumlocution response made when someone cannot retrieve the phonological representation (form) of a word, but can find semantic information so gives a description of the meaning of a word, e.g. 'knife' – you use it to cut things.

Compensation strategies these aim to use remaining language skills and communication abilities as strategies to communicate rather than working to improve damaged language functions.

Competence refers to our knowledge of language, distinct from our ability with language (**performance**) which may be limited by e.g. aphasia.

Conduite d'approche repeated attempts to say a word, making phonological errors, often getting closer to the target word. This may point to difficulties with phonological assembly.

Content words convey most of the meaning of a sentence and can be nouns, adjectives, verbs or adverbs.

CVA cerebral vascular accident or stroke involving a blockage or rupture of a blood vessel in the brain, leading to damage to the surrounding brain tissue.

Deep dysgraphia a writing disorder where someone finds some words easier to write than others; concrete words better than abstract words, content words better than function words. They cannot write nonwords and make semantic and visual errors in writing.

Deep dyslexia a reading disorder with semantic substitution errors, e.g. 'dog' is read as 'cat', 'smile' is read as 'happy'; visual errors, e.g. 'fire' is read as 'fine'; poor nonword reading, and word class affects reading (e.g. concrete words are read more accurately than abstract words, and there are more difficulties with function words than with content words).

Discourse chunks of language involving several sentences, e.g. a monologue or dialogue.

Dissociation when someone with aphasia has impairment in one language area and not in another, e.g. they may not understand words when they are written but can understand the same words when spoken.

Dysarthria a motor speech disorder involving slower and weaker movements of the muscles needed to produce both speech and voice.

Dyscalculia impairment of number and mathematical skills; of calculation, reading and writing numbers.

Dysgraphia a writing disorder.

Dyslexia a reading disorder.

Dysphagia a swallowing disorder.

Expressive to do with the production (of language).

Facilitate make processing information quicker, opposite of inhibit.

Function words do the grammatical work in a sentence, e.g. prepositions, conjunctions and determiners.

Global aphasia refers to aphasia where there is significant impairment in all language modalities.

Grapheme a letter or letter group corresponding to a phoneme.

Graphemic output buffer a store of graphemic representations or letters (including upper- and lower-case forms).

Graphemic output lexicon a store of the forms of known written words or how they are spelled.

Graphic motor programming translating letter forms to motor patterns to write words.

Handedness 95 per cent of right-handed people and about 75 per cent of left-handed people have language processing dominant in the left hemisphere. Most left-handed people with aphasia have had left hemisphere lesions. They may present with similar language difficulties after a stroke, or there may be more variability in language characteristics and in recovery as they may have some language representation in both cerebral hemispheres, which can aid recovery.

Hemianopia a visual field deficit with a loss of vision for stimuli in the visual field opposite the site of the brain lesion (contralesional).

Hemiparesis a muscle weakness in the side of the body opposite the site of the brain lesion.

Hemiplegia   paralysis affecting one side of the body, when the lesion is above the level of the brain stem it is on the opposite side to the hemisphere where the brain lesion occurred. As aphasia usually follows damage in the left hemisphere, there is usually a right hemiplegia.

Hemisphere   the brain is divided into two halves or hemispheres, left and right.

Inhibit   to slow down the processing of information, also refers to suppressing unwanted options, e.g. refers to the way connections in language networks reduce activation of units.

Inner speech   language we hear internally but is not articulated as speech.

Jargon   spontaneous speech where most words produced are nonwords or neologisms so the listener derives little meaning from it. There may be real word production, but it is often unrelated to an appropriate target.

Lesion   a brain lesion is an area of brain tissue that shows damage from injury or disease.

Lexicon   the set of words in someone's vocabulary, their mental dictionary.

Logogen   is a specialised recognition unit or module that doesn't contain the word itself but the phonemic and graphemic information about a word. The information can be used to recognise and/or retrieve the word. When we hear or read a word, the logogen for that word is activated. Logogen models suggest a way of thinking about how language is understood and produced.

Minimal pair   a pair of words, with different meanings, where only one sound in the word is changed, e.g. 'cat' and 'bat' or 'send' and 'mend'.

Modelling   is a term used in behavioural therapy to describe the way the clinician provides the client with an example of how to do something which they can copy or imitate to achieve production.

Module/modular   viewing cognitive functions as independent processes that can be separately damaged or intact. See *logogen*.

Neglect   an attention deficit where someone may not respond appropriately to stimuli (visual, auditory or tactile) presented at the side opposite the site of the lesion.

Neologisms word errors in spontaneous speech that are non-words (less than 50 per cent of the sounds in the target word are in the nonword produced).

Neuron a nerve cell.

Nonword a string of letters or sounds that do not make up a word, e.g. 'crid' or 'cosp'.

Orthographic input lexicon a store of the forms of written words that someone has in their vocabulary.

Orthographic output lexicon a store of these familiar written words with their spelling.

Orthographic-to-phonological conversion (non-lexical reading route) reading aloud by sounding out the letters of a word rather than reading via the lexicon or word store.

Orthography the written form and spelling of words.

Paraphasia a spoken word substitution. Phonemic or formal paraphasias are similar in their phonological form to the target word; phonemes may be omitted, substituted or moved within the word and other sounds may be added but at least 50 per cent of the phonemes of the target word are included, e.g., calling a dog, a 'dot', or it could result in a nonword, so 'dog' becomes 'gog'. An example of a semantic paraphasia, where the substitution is made following the meaning of the word, might be to call a 'dog', a 'wolf'.

Perseveration repeating a previous response to a new stimulus. Verbal perseverations may be the inappropriate repetition of a previous response that was correct/incorrect. Perseverations reflect the underlying language deficits, usually word retrieval problems, so treatment is via appropriate aphasia therapy, i.e. to treat the word retrieval difficulties. It is particularly prevalent in the first three months post onset of the aphasia but can persist. Management includes dealing with the frustration it can cause to the person with aphasia and their family via education and strategies. These can include longer pauses/silence to allow the perseverative response to weaken.

Phoneme the smallest sound used in language.

Phoneme-to-grapheme conversion (non-lexical writing route) rather than writing the whole word by accessing the word store, this route involves breaking a word up into sounds and converting the sounds into letters.

Phonemic cueing giving a phonological (sound) cue to help someone say a word; usually the first phoneme and then gradually more phonological information.

Phonological assembly a stage in spoken word production where sounds are selected and put together in the appropriate order to make up the chosen word.

Phonological dysgraphia a spelling disorder where real word spelling is better than nonword spelling (damage to the connection between the phonological-to-graphemic conversion modules).

Phonological errors are errors that are similar to the phonological form of the target word (they share at least 50 per cent of the phonemes).

Phonological input lexicon is where auditory word recognition units are stored and from where the words someone hears can be recognised as familiar. A deficit here can lead to word form deafness. Where there is a disruption to the link between this lexicon and the semantic system, there can be word meaning deafness.

Phonological output lexicon spoken word forms are stored and can be accessed from here.

Phonology sounds, the study of sounds and how they are used in language.

Pragmatics includes skills beyond just meanings of words, e.g. choice of words, understanding implications of word choices in conversation and maintaining topic coherence.

Priming either facilitating or inhibiting a response to what you are presenting, by by showing something semantically or phonologically related to it beforehand. Semantic priming helps produce a word similar in meaning, e.g. plate -> bowl.

Psycholinguistic variables these are aspects of words that can affect the performance of someone with aphasia, e.g. regularly spelled and irregularly spelled words are significant factors for people with reading and writing deficits. Other variables that have an impact on language processing in aphasia include word length, imageability, frequency and age-of-acquisition.

Letter-by-letter reading difficulties recognising and reading a word unless each individual letter is identified by name. Sometimes there are errors involving letters that are visually similar. Where someone has good writing alongside these reading difficulties, it may be called **pure alexia.**

Reactivation approach   an approach that focuses on regaining access to impaired language and language processing through therapy that reactivates that processing.

Receptive   refers to comprehension of language and is used to describe an aphasia where the main difficulty seems to be comprehension rather than expression of language.

Relearning approach   to therapy reteaches impaired language.

Semantic cueing   giving semantic information (e.g. meanings or related meanings) to help someone produce a word.

Semantic error   a response that is semantically related to the target word, e.g. .'comb' -> 'brush'.

Semantic feature   something that represents part of the meaning of a word.

Semantic lexical route for reading   this involves accessing the meaning of a word when reading aloud.

Semantic lexical route for writing   this involves accessing the meaning of a word when writing

Semantic memory a   memory system with long-term store of facts/knowledge of the world, e.g. an owl is a bird.

Semantic system   a store of word meanings.

Short term memory   (STM) see *working memory.*

Surface dysgraphia   involves generally good spelling of words that follow regular spelling patterns ('regular' words such as 'dog' and nonwords) but difficulties spelling irregular words (e.g. 'sew' may be written as 'so').

Surface dyslexia   involves fairly intact reading of regular and nonwords (e.g. 'new') but difficulty reading irregular words, e.g. 'sew'. A person with surface dyslexia has difficulty accessing the orthographic input lexicon. Using the phonological-to-graphemic conversion route they may produce a possible version of a word, e.g. 'bear' may be read aloud as 'beer'.

Thematic roles   the semantic roles in a sentence, conveying information about who is doing what to whom (e.g. agent) rather than syntactic roles (e.g. object).

Tip-of-the-tongue   (TOT) describes the experience of knowing a word but being unable to access it in speech, even while being aware of the first sound or letter of the word.

Visual error   errors made in reading where the error is similar to the target word in its orthographic form (e.g. the word 'hand' read as 'band').

Visual orthographic analysis   this is where letters are identified and their position in a word is processed.

Working memory   or short-term memory (STM) is a limited memory for recent events. When we look at digit span, for example, we are looking at the STM ability to hold information for a few minutes, such as telephone numbers.

INDEX

Note: For figure citations, page numbers appear in *italics*.

A-FROM model 3, 20–1, 38, 128, 135, 175, 183, 189–90; framework for outcome measurement diagram *203*
AAC *see* augmentative and alternative communication (AAC)
ABI *see* acquired brain injury (ABI)
acalculia: definition 236
access to services 181–2
acquired brain injury (ABI) 4, 7, 12, 34, 99, 175–6, 190, 213, 230; advice 91; aphasia management 45; attention deficits 92; definition 236; treatment 91
atrophy 236
activities of daily living (ADL) 8, 65
activity 16, 19
acute: ABI 45; aphasia management 2, 40–6; COVID-19 infection 93; hospitals 39, 40, 43–5; recovery stage 39, 122, 206–7; strokes 12, 26; therapy 42, 135
Adult Carers Quality of Life questionnaire (Ac-QOL) 38, 219
advocacy 44, 117–18
agrammatism: definition 236
agraphia: definition 236

alexia *see* pure alexia
Alzheimer's dementia (AD) 8–9, 13, 46, 175; *see also* dementia
American Speech-Language-Hearing Association (ASHA) Quality of Communication Life Quality of Communication Life Scale (ASHA QCL) 219
aneurysm 6
anomia 131, 161; definition 236
anomic aphasia 15
anoxia 6–7; definition 236
anoxic brain injury 7, 12; *see also* brain injury
antidepressants 187, 192
anxiety 6, 30, 179, 181, 184–5; linguistic 184, 190; mindfulness and 193; post-stroke 192; professional support for 194
Aphasia Centre 117, 177
Aphasia Impact Questionnaire 38, 210
Aphasia Institute 38, 66, 81, *203*, 229–30; free online e-learning: Supported Conversation for Adults with Aphasia (SCA™); Pictographic Resources folder 211–12
aphasia management 25–59; acute stage 40–5; barriers 40; pressures 39

Aphasia Screening Test 211
Aphasia Scripts 155
Aphasia Severity Rating (ASR) 210
Aphasia Software Finder 156
Aphasia Support (UK) 227, 234
Aphasia Therapy Finder 230–1
Aphasia Therapy Online 234
approaches: choice of 21; understanding aphasia 11–24
apps 101, 154–6
Apraxia Battery for Adults (ABA) 100
apraxia of speech (AOS) 2, 99–102; assessment 100–1; other apraxias compared 101; treatment 100–2; *see also* limb apraxia; oral apraxia
argument structure: definition 236
art therapy 192
articulate, articulatory programming: definition 236
assessment 2, 60–85, 88–91, 210–25; aphasia management 40–1; apraxia of speech (AOS) 100–1; attention 89; baselines 60–1; common issues 77–81; comprehension 78; COVID-19 pandemic 94; cut-off for 80; diagnosis 60; dysarthria 103; fact finding mission 80; formal 71; getting everything 'wrong' 80; goal setting 60–1; impact of 76–7; informal 63–4; management 60; memory 89–90; neglect 89; observations 64–5; options 63; outcome measures 61; post-assessment 82; preparation for 62; rationale for 60–2; reporting on 82; self-preparation 62; standardised 71; structured format 73; therapy 61–2; time for 81 treatment options 60; well-being 189–91
associated communication disorders: clinical diagnosis 99–108
Association for Speech & Language Therapists in Independent Practice (ASLTIP) 227
ataxic dysarthria *see* dysarthria
atherosclerosis 6
atrophy: definition 236
attention 87–8, 135, 212; assessment of 89; deficits 87, 92, 105; difficulties 5; visual therapy 92; *see also* hemianopia; neglect
auditory comprehension 135–6
auditory phonological analysis: definition 236
Augmentative and Alternative Communication (AAC) 43, 48, 104, 138, 140–1, 206–7, 234; appropriate level 141; clear instructions 141; personalisation 141; practice 141
autobiographical memory interview 218
autoimmune encephalitis 7
automatic speech: definition 236
avoidance 181, 190–1
awareness: aphasia patients 65, 67, 79; grammatical 137; metacognition 92 public 181–3, 228; self-awareness 176, 179

balance *see* recovery
barriers 146–50, 230; assessment 40; to communication 16, 20, 36, 45, 181–2; technological 154
baselines: assessment 60–1; definition 237
BDAE 214

INDEX

BDAE-3 217
best practice 25
Better Conversations with Aphasia 49, 234
Better Conversations with PPA (BCPPA) 49
bilingualism: clients 214; factors 49–51; interpreters 50–1
Bitsboard 234
body functions and structures 16
Boston Naming Test 214, 217
Boston School 15
brain: approaches to aphasia 12–13; bleeding 6, 12; cerebral cortex 11–12; cerebrum 11; injury *see* brain injury; lesions 4–5; lesions 183; neural network 13–14 ; scans 14–15; stimulation 2, 109–10; trauma *see* brain trauma; tumours *see* brain tumours; understanding 11–12; vascular system 12
brain injury: anoxic 7, 12; causes of 7; education 188–9; metabolic/toxic 7; *see also* acquired brain injury (ABI)
brain trauma 4, 205
brain tumour 2, 4, 8, 12, 39–40, 176, 205; cancerous and non-cancerous 8; surgical interventions 8; treatments 8; types of 8
British Aphasiology Society (BAS) 39, 231
Broca, Paul 4
Broca's aphasia 15–16, 72

cancer 175
carers: support for 49
CAT *see* Comprehensive Aphasia Test (CAT)
CAT/CT scans (computerised tomography/computerised axial tomogram) 14
causes of aphasia 4–10; importance of 4–5
cerebral vascular accident (CVA) 4–7; definition 237
charities 180
chronic: ABI 45; aphasia management 2, 46, 122; conditions 179, 180; recovery stage 39, 40, 42, 206–7
circumlocution 30, 132; definition 237
City Gesture Checklist 212
CIU Analysis 214
classification systems 15–16
client discussion 21–2
clinical diagnosis: associated communication disorders 99–108
clinical excellence networks (CENs) 39
clinical guidelines 25, 208, 209, 226–7
clinical psychologists 188
clinical supervisors 194–5
Cochrane Review 125
cognition: language and 17, 86–7
cognitive assessments 216
cognitive communication disorders 93
cognitive deficits 91
cognitive functions 212
cognitive impairments 2, 86–98; treatment 91–3
Cognitive Linguistic Quick Test (CLQT) 212, 216
cognitive neuropsychology 17, 19
cognitive-communication disorders 2
Collaboration of Aphasia Trialists (CATS) 230, 232

colleagues 194
Communication Effectiveness Index (CETI) 38, 210
communication partners 147, 207
communication support 48
community organisations 154, 180–1
compensation claims: for medical negligence 116
compensation strategies: definition 237
compensatory therapy 2, 95, 120, 127, 137–42, 160–2, 207; dysarthria 104
competence: definition 237; *see also* performance
comprehension: assessment of 78–9, 213; auditory 16, 36, 87–8, 122, 135–6, 161, 215, 217; conservational strategies 146; deficit 101; difficulties 41, 62, 78–9, 86, 135, 139, 141, 145, 158–61; discourse 91; education 43; language 47, 72, 103, 215, 242; in PPA 47; reading 15, 61, 88; semantic therapies for 135; sentence 73, 130, 132–4, 215, 236; signs/object-to-picture matching 219; spoken 124; verb 161; word 132; written 15, 100, 145, 153
Comprehensive Aphasia Test (CAT) 37–9, 72, 81, 94, 134, 214–15; Cognitive Screen section 212; Language Battery 210
computer therapy 101, 122, 141, 154–6, 207; digital divide 154; disabled users 154
conduction aphasia 15
conduite d'approche 132; definition 237

Connect (organisation) 227; ideas series 232
connections: building 1–2; cerebral 29; language networks 239; language processing 17–18; making 114; mapping therapy 134–5; neural 1, 236; neural plasticity 28; social 128, 152, 155
consequences of aphasia 19
constraint induced aphasia therapy (CIAT) 136, 146, 150
content words: definition 237
conversation 66–71, 207; assessing 213; communication difficulties 67–70; discourse 70–1; errors 32–3; everyday talk 64; 'good' 32; narrative 70–1; partner training 148, 220; resources 232; speech recordings 69–70, 144–6; support for 69–70, 144–6; supported 29, 43, 145–6, 177, 185; tender 186; turn-taking 68, 74, 105; written samples 71
Conversation Analysis Profile for People with Aphasia (CAPPA) 213
Conversation Analysis Profile for People with Cognitive Impairment (CAPCI) 212
Cookie Theft picture 77, 217
Copy and Recall Treatment (CART) 133
counselling 192, 195, 201; education 191; management 40, 44; reading suggestions 201; skills 188, 191; training in 188
COVID-19 pandemic 93–5, 156; assessment 94; delivery 95; Long Covid/post COVID condition 93–4; post-COVID

condition 2; referral 94; therapy 94–5
crossed aphasia 105
cueing: hierarchies 130; *see also* phonemic cueing; semantic cueing
CueSpeak 234
CVA *see* cerebral vascular accident (CVA)

damage: diffuse 4; focal 4
deafness: word form/word sound 135, 241
deep dysgraphia: definition 237
deep dyslexia: definition 237
deficits: attention 92; cognitive 91
delivery (of therapy) 95, 157–8, 207; options 2, 150–4; speech delivery 156; Telehealth 156
dementia 4, 8–9, 13, 46, 78, 93–4, 231; atrophy 236; mixed 9; *see also* Alzheimer's dementia (AD); semantic dementia (SD); vascular dementia (VaD)
Dementia with Lewy bodies (DLB) 8, 46
depression 177, 179, 181, 183–4
Depression Intensity Scale Circles (DISCs) 38, 213
devices, digital 141
diadochokinetic rate 100
diagnosis 41; assessment 60; differential 60
dignity 205
disability 175, 177; language 5; terminological use 190
discharge 37, 45, 105, 123
discourse 105; assessing 213–14; conversation and 70–1; definition 237
disorder of the person 184
dissociation: definition 238
drawing 69, 140
drawing attention to aphasia 92–3
dysarthria 2, 94, 102–4; assessment 103; ataxic 12, 103–4; behavioural treatment 104; compensatory therapy 104; definition 238; flaccid 102; functional interventions 104; hyperkinetic 103; hypokinetic 103–4; mixed 103; spastic 102–3; treatment 104; types of 102–3; unilateral upper motor neuron 102
dyscalculia 212; definition 238
Dyscover (organisation) 228, 234
dysgraphia: definition 236, 238; *see also* deep dysgraphia; phonological dysgraphia; surface dysgraphia
dyslexia 17; definition 238; *see also* deep dyslexia; surface dyslexia
dysphagia 39–40, 45, 126–7; definition 238

education 43–5: about aphasia 31, 91, 153; brain injury 188–9; on recovery 27–8
Egypt, ancient 4
Eliot, George 3
embolism 6
emergencies 74
emotion 187, 193; emotional lability 13; emotional well-being *see* well-being
end-of-life care 40, 208
ending therapy *see* discharge
English as a second language (ESL) 50
environment 16, 19
environmental adaptation 2, 180–1
environmental intervention 207

environmental therapy 95
Equality Act (UK) 22n1
errors: apraxia of speech 100; bilingualism 51; conversational 32–3; learning 31; phonological 132; word 132; *see also* semantic error; phonological errors; visual error
executive functions 87, 105, 135, 212
exercise 179
expertise, sharing 116–17
experts 115–16
explaining aphasia 60–1
expressive: definition 238

FaceTime 150, 156
facilitate: definition 238
family: group therapy, involvement in 151; impact on 2, 177–8; support for families 49, 207; talking with 195
fatigue 95, 183, 189
financial stability 179
flaccid dysarthria *see* dysarthria
fMRI (functional magnetic resonance imaging) 14, 29, 109
foreign accent syndrome 94
formal assessments of language comprehension and production 213
Frenchay Aphasia Screening Test (FAST) 211, 216
friends 178, 181; peer befriending 149–50; support 49; talking with 195
Frontotemporal lobar degeneration (FTD/FTLD) 9, 13, 46–7
frustration 68–9, 90, 94, 112, 177, 183–5

function words: definition 238
functional communication 73–4, 216–17
Functional Linguistic Communication Inventory (FLCI-2) 218–19
functional/participation-oriented therapy 207

generalisation 12, 48, 121, 133, 135, 149, 155; therapy gains 158–62
gesture 49, 69, 101, 124, 139–40, 148, 157, 212; production assessment test 218; training 102
global aphasia 15–16, 135; definition 238
goal setting 29–32, 41–2
goals 38, 121–3, 153, 176; assessment of 63, 76, 82; clients 3, 20, 21, 127, 129, 151; communication 150, 227; conversational 152, 161; discharge 37; flexibility of 48; functional 149; interviews on 65; motivation and 32–3; return to work 34; setting 29–32, 41–2, 61
Graded Naming Test 217
grapheme: definition 238
graphemic output buffer a: definition 238
graphemic output lexicon: definition 238
graphic motor programming: definition 238
grief reaction 183–4
group therapy 33, 49, 91, 150–4, 158, 177–8, 207; education about aphasia 153; family involvement 151; home practice 153; non-verbal communication 152; participation 152

group treatment 150
guidelines: clinical 25, 39, 40, 42, 49, 125, 226–7; stroke 206

haemorrhagic stroke *see* stroke
handedness: definition 238
HEADS: UP Aphasia Helping Ease Anxiety and Depression Following Stroke 193
Headway 226
Health Care and Professions Council (HCPC) 194
health care professionals 82
health insurance 37, 81
hemianopia: attention 88; definition 238
hemiplegia 154; definition 239
hemisphere: definition 239; language-dominant 4; *see also* right hemisphere disorders
historical approaches 4
hobbies 65, 70, 153, 183
hopelessness 184
Hue camera 157
human connection 114–15
human rights, respect for 205–6
humour *see* black humour
Huntington's disease 103
hyperkinetic dysarthria *see* dysarthria
hypertension 6
hypokinetic dysarthria *see* dysarthria
hypoxia: definition 236

ICAPs *see* Intensive Comprehensive Aphasia Programs (ICAPs)
iceberg metaphor 190
ideational apraxia 139, 212
identity: reconstruction 188; theft 188

ideomotor apraxia 139, 212
impact of aphasia 60–1; on family 2, 177–8; individuals 2, 175–7; psychological 2–3, 183
impairment 21, 61, 104, 238; cognitive 2, 13, 46, 86–95, 117; communication 8, 20, 40, 146, 184; language 2, 16–17, 19, 37–8, 60, 70–3, 128, 131, 150, 205, 210, 214–15; measurement of 37–8
impairment-based treatment 2, 49, 120, 122, 127–8, 144–5, 149, 161–2, 207, 217; semantic approach 140, 160; therapeutic examples 131–8, 207; tools 217
independence: loss of 183
informal assessments 211–12
inhibit: definition 239
inner speech: definition 239
intelligence 205
Intensive Comprehensive Aphasia Programme @ Queen Square 228
Intensive Comprehensive Aphasia Programs (ICAPs) 126, 149, 159
interactive activation models 18
Intercollegiate Stroke Working Party 226, 227
International Best Practice Recommendations for Aphasia 205–9; preamble 205–6; primary sources 208–9; top ten recommendations 206–8
interviews 211; semi-structured interactive 65–6
intonation 105
intracerebral haemorrhage 6
intracranial haematoma 7
iPads 141, 154, 160
ischaemic stroke *see* stroke

jargon 124; definition 239

Kabat-Zinn, J. 193
Kagan, A. 66, 112, 217

language: cognition and 17, 86–7; loss of 183–4; translation issues 49–50; use 105; world languages 1; *see also* bilingualism
language impairment 71–3
language performance: assessments of 217–19
language processing 2, 60, 73 model 3, 17–19, *204*
learned non-use of speech 146
learning 130–1; cueing hierarchies 130; errors 131; feedback 130–1; with aphasia 131
Lee Silverman Voice Treatment (LSVT®) 104
legal cases 116
lesion(s): definition 239; location of 26; size 26
letter-by-letter reading: definition 241–2
lexical-semantic processing 105
lexicon: definition 239
life expectancy 5, 176
Life Interests and Values cards 211
Life Participation Approach in Aphasia (LPAA) 20–1, 149, 152, 228, 231
limb apraxia 13, 100, 139, 218, 101
lip-reading 145, 156
listening 186
living well 2, 178–80
living with aphasia 175–201
logogen: definition 239; model 18, *204*, 239
logopenic progressive aphasia (LPA) 13, 47

loneliness 184–5
LPAA *see* Life Participation Approach in Aphasia (LPAA)

M-MAT *see* Multi-modality Aphasia Therapy (M-MAT)
management *see* aphasia management
medical issues 25
medical training 182
medication 2, 110
meditation 179, 192–3
melodic intonation therapy (MIT) 101
memory 88, 212; assessment of 89–90; difficulties 5; non-verbal episodic 105; nonverbal recognition 212; strokes 13; treatments 91; *see also* short-term memory (STM); working memory (WM)
meningitis 7
Mental Capacity Act (UK) 117
mental health: conditions 192; emergency teams 187; services 182, 192
Mental Health Trust 191
middle cerebral artery (MCA) 12
mild aphasia 77
mind-body practices 192; *see also* meditation; mindfulness
mindfulness 192–3
Mindfulness based stress reduction (MBSR) 193
minimal pair: definition 239; discrimination 135
mixed dysarthria *see* dysarthria
Mixed Transcortical aphasia 15
mobility loss 183
modality charts 138
modelling: definition 239

models 21, 69, 92, 126, 129–30, 133, 140; A-FROM 3, 20–1, 38; brain 12; conversations 148, 186; gestures 139; group therapy 150; language processing 3, 17–19, 72–3, 128, *204*; role model 153; social 149, 190
module/modular: definition 239
mood 177; disorders 192; measurements of 38; regulation 183, 188; *see also* well-being
motivation 32–3, 48
motor neuron disease (MND) 103
MRI (magnetic resonance imaging) 14, 29
multi-disciplinary teams (MDTs) 44, 89, 115
Multi-modality Aphasia Therapy (M-MAT) 122, 143–4, 146
multimodal communication 37, 122, 145, 149, 157
multiple sclerosis (MS) 103
music therapy 192; *see also* melodic intonation therapy (MIT)
Myerson, Debra 179–80

narrative therapy 161; *see also* conversation
National Institute for Health and Care Excellence (NICE) 226; Clinical Guidelines 42, 49
National Institute for Health and Care Research (NIHR) 226–7
nature of aphasia 60
neglect: assessment of 89; attention 87; definition 239; treatment 92; unilateral 87; visual 88, 105, 212
neologisms: definition 240
neural networks 18, 128
neural plasticity 2, 28–9

neuroimaging 18; brain's neural network 13–14 ; studies 29, 122
neuron a: definition 240
neuroplasticity 110, 125, 128
neurorehabilitation units 45
Newcastle University Aphasia Therapy Resources 134
NHS (National Health Service) 45–6
NICE Clinical Guidelines *see* National Institute for Health and Care Excellence (NICE)
Non-invasive brain stimulation (NIBS) 109
non-lexical reading route *see* orthographic-to-phonological conversion
non-lexical writing route *see* phoneme-to-grapheme conversion
non-verbal communication 152
nonword: definition 240
North East Trust for Aphasia (NETA) 228, 235

occupational therapists 102, 188
oedema (swelling) 6–7
Office for National Statistics (ONS) 52n1
online groups 234
onset of aphasia: severity 26–7; time since 27
oral apraxia 100–1
oral reading 101
Oral Reading for Language in Aphasia (ORLA) 155
organisations 180, 227–9
orthographic analysis *see* visual orthographic analysis
orthographic input lexicon a: definition 240
orthographic output lexicon: definition 240

orthographic-to-phonological conversion: definition 240
orthography: definition 240
outcomes: measurement of 37–8

PACE *see* Promoting Aphasic Communicative Effectiveness (PACE)
PALPA *see* Psycholinguistic Assessment of Language Processing in Aphasia (PALPA)
paralysis 64, 154, 183
paraphasia: definition 240
paresis 64
Parkinson's disease (PD) 8–9, 46, 103–4
participation 16, 19
Participation in Life Situations and Communication and Language Environment 135–6
peer supervision 194
performance: definition 237; *see also* competence
perseveration: definition 240
personal animated therapist (PAT) 155
personality traits 179, 189
perspective 136–7
PET (positron emission tomography) 15
pharmacotherapy 110
phone calls 30
phoneme: definition 240
phoneme-to-grapheme conversion: definition 240
phonemic cueing: definition 241
phonological assembly: definition 241
phonological components analysis (PCA) 133
phonological dysgraphia: definition 241
phonological errors: definition 241

phonological input lexicon: definition 241
phonological output lexicon: definition 241
phonology: definition 241
physiological consequences of aphasia 183–5
physiotherapists 102
plasticity *see* neural plasticity; neuroplasticity
PLORAS 29
PPA *see* primary progressive aphasia (PPA)
pragmatics 105; definition 241
primary progressive aphasia (PPA) 9, 37, 46–9; assessment in 48; diagnosis 48; extended 47; goals 48; monitoring 48; non-fluent variant PPA (nfvPPA) 47; optimisation 48; semantic (PPA-S) 47; semantic variant PPA (svPPA) 47; SLT management of 47–8; therapy 48–9; types of 13; *see also* logopenic progressive aphasia (LPA)
priming: definition 241
processing speed 88; testing 90
prognosis 25–8, 41, 60–1
progressive aphasia 2, 9, 46–7, 176; management of 46–9; *see also* primary progressive aphasia (PPA)
progressive non-fluent aphasia (PNFA) 13, 47
Promoting Aphasic Communicative Effectiveness (PACE) 142, 160
prosody 100, 103, 105
prosopagnosia 105
psychiatry 189, 191–2
Psycholinguistic Assessment of Language Processing in Aphasia (PALPA) 19, 72, 214–15

psycholinguistic variables: definition 241
psychological consequences 183–5; *see also* anxiety; depression
psychological impact of aphasia 2–3, 183
psychological issues: addressing 185–9; asking questions 185–9
psychological treatments 191–3
psychology 192
psychotherapy 192
public awareness of aphasia 181–3
pure alexia: definition 242
Pyramids and Palm Trees 72, 217

quadriplegia 175
quality of life (QOL) 5, 38, 61, 86, 175, 219
Quick Aphasia Battery (QAB) 211

ramps 146–50
rating scales 210–11
reactivation approach: definition 242
reading 14, 16, 34, 65, 80; ability 135; aloud 48, 100, 215, 240; comprehension 15, 36, 61, 88, 159; difficulties 47, 62, 92, 93, 155, 214, 241, 242; disorders 237–8, 241–2; lip 104, 145, 156; memory treatments 91; oral 101; scans 5; visual neglect 105
receptive: definition 242
recovery 25–8; balance 27–8; education 27–8; encouragement 27–8; key factors predicting 26–7; pace of 28; reading suggestions 53–4; spontaneous 25; understanding of 25
rehabilitation 22, 75, 102, 153, 177, 193
relationships 1, 16, 66, 183, 191; A-FROM model *203*; conversations, importance of 144; negative impact on 175, 177, 179, 205; personal experiences of 115
relearning approach: definition 242
repetition 15, 22, 28, 31, 48, 100, 101, 126, 128–130, 133, 143, 145 150, 159, 162, 190, 215, 240
resources 39, 50, 63, 76, 121, 226–35; pictographic 211; psychological 179; therapeutic 129; video 157
respect 205
return to work 25, 33–6, 65, 95
right hemisphere disorders 105
Royal College of Speech and Language Therapists (RCSLT) 116, 118n1, 227

safeguarding 186–7
Scanning Eye training as a Rehabilitation Choice for Hemianopia after stroke (SEARCH) 95
scanning pens 155
scans 5, 14–15, 92, 95n1
Scenario Test 37, 213
screening tests 211
scripts 158; practice 155; training 144
self-development 193–5
self-disclosure 144
self-esteem 33
self-regulation strategies 192
semantic cueing: definition 242
semantic dementia (SD) 13, 47
semantic error: definition 242

semantic feature: definition 242
semantic feature analysis (SFA) 132–3
semantic lexical route for reading: definition 242
semantic lexical route for writing: definition 242
semantic memory: access to 212; definition 242
semantic system: definition 242
semantic therapy 135
sentence(s): completion 130, 132; comprehension 135–6, 215; discourse 237; errors 51, 113; function words 238; incomplete 160; level difficulties 42, 48, 70; processing 30, 131, 133–5, 186; production 21, 47, 113, 122, 152, 155; repetition 91, 131; shorter 104; structures 137, 236; thematic roles 242; written comprehension 73
Sentence Production Treatment 155
Sentence Shaper 234
severe aphasia 80–1
severity of aphasia 60; at onset 26–7
SFA Therapy resource 231
short-term memory (STM) 88, 91, 243; definition 242
small talk 114
software 2, 154–6, 234; Aphasia Software Finder 229, 234; speech to text 154–5; text to speech 155
spastic dysarthria *see* dysarthria
Speakeasy 228
speaking: thinking for 136–7
speaking valve placement 45
speech and language therapists (SLTs) 1, 5, 28, 34; acute sector 40; bilingualism, challenges of 50; community input 45; counselling skills 188, 191; effectiveness of 110; financial constraints 37; gestures 139; interactive approach 66; management pressures 39; one-to-one input 44; PPA management 47–8; professional support for 194–5; role of 114; transcribing conversations 71; *see also* therapists
speech recordings 71; *see also* conversation
Speech Sounds on Cue 101, 234
spontaneous recovery *see* recovery
stammering 94, 190
strategies 78, 120, 128; communication 32, 48–9, 51, 69, 87, 123–4, 152; compensatory 146–7, 162, 237; conversational 28, 39, 51, 79, 143, 145, 148, 158; development of 191–3; learning 121; memory 91; metacognitive 91–2; multimodal 122, 138, 145, 149; non-verbal and verbal 21; self-regulation 192; teaching 115; training with 102; types of 30–1, 43, 104, 140–3
stress 184, 193–4
stroke 2, 5–7, 207; atrophy 236; brain lesions 4; family history of 6; haemorrhagic 5–6, 27; ischaemic 5, 27; memory of 13; risk factors 6
Stroke and Aphasia Handbook (it) 178
Stroke Association (UK) 193, 228
subacute stage 40
suicidal ideation 187

support: carers 49; communication 48; communication partners 44; family 49; friends 49; impairment-based 48; psychological 183, 191–3; strategies 48
surface dysgraphia: definition 242
surface dyslexia: definition 242
swallowing problems 81; *see also* dysphagia

Tactus ® Apps 92, 101
Talking Mats 118
talking therapies 192; *see also* counselling
Tavistock Aphasia Centre 126, 228
Tavistock Trust for Aphasia 229
TBI *see* traumatic brain injury (TBI)
technology aids 104, 141
telehealth 2, 150, 156–8; on delivery 157–8
telerehabilitation 207
text messaging (SMS) 156
thematic roles: definition 242
therapeutic relationship 2, 112
therapists 111–19; confidence 112; interactions 113; making connections 114; qualities 111; supportive environment 112; talking to 195; *see also* Speech and Language Therapists (SLTs)
therapy 2, 27, 120–74; acute and subacute stages 42; amount of 42–3; approaches to 127–8; assessment and 61–2; assessment as part of 74–6; barriers and ramps 146–50; behavioural 120; client-centred 114; combining 159–62; computer programs/apps 101, 122, 141, 154–6; COVID-19 pandemic 94–5; definition of 120; delivery options 2, 150–4; ending *see* discharge; environmental 95; evidence for 28, 42–3, 50, 61, 91, 92, 110, 120, 122, 125, 126, 131, 133, 155, 192, 230; functioning 122–4; gains, generalisation of 158–9; gains, maintaining 159; goals 180; group 33, 49, 91, 150–4, 158, 177–8, 207; intensity/dose of 125–6; intensive programmes 122; key steps 120–2; Life Participation 20, 63, 149, 237; longevity of 125–6; mapping 134–5; phonological 30, 122, 133, 160, 162; provisional limitations 126–7; repetition 128–9; resources for clients 233; resources for clinicians 230–3; semantic 132, 135, 161; types of 42; words for 137; writing 133; *see also* compensatory therapy; computer therapy; impairment-based treatment
Therapy Outcome Measure (TOM) 38
thinking for speaking 136–7
third-party functioning 177
TIA (transient ischaemic attack) 6
tip-of-the-tongue (TOT): definition 242
Total Communication 43, 122, 124, 138, 142–4, 146, 160; AAC and 141; drawing 140; group therapy 152
Tourette's syndrome 103
tracheostomy 45

INDEX   257

Transcortical Motor aphasia 15
Transcortical Sensory
  aphasia 15
transcranial direct current
  stimulation (tDCS) 109
transcranial magnetic
  stimulation (TMS) 109;
  repetitive (rTMS) 109
traumatic brain injury (TBI)
  7, 39; dysarthria 102–3;
  memory and 88; processing
  speed and 88
treatment 109–10; appropriate
  type and amount of 27;
  apraxia of speech (AOS)
  100–2; brain stimulation 109;
  brain tumour 8; cognitive
  impairments 91–3; dysarthria
  104, impairment-based 128;
  medication 110; memory 91;
  options 60; psychological
  191–3
triangle model 18
tumours see brain tumours

ultrasound 101
understanding aphasia 60

vascular cognitive impairment
  (VCI) 13
Vascular dementia (VaD) 8–3,
  13, 46; see also dementia
  verb and sentence processing
  133–4
Verb Network Strengthening
  Treatment (VNeST) 48,
  134, 216
Very Early Rehabilitation in
  Speech (VERSE) 42
videoconferencing 156
viral encephalitis 103
Visual Analogue Self Esteem
  Scale (VASES) 211, 214

visual attention therapy 92
visual-auditory recognition 212
visual error: definition 243
visual orthographic analysis:
  definition 243
visual scanning training 92
visual-spatial abilities 212
visualisers 157

walking sticks 64
websites 3, 226–35
Webster, J. 134
well-being 153, 177; assessment
  of 189–91; emotional,
  assessment of 214
Wernicke, Carl 4
Wernicke's aphasia 15, 72
Western Aphasia Battery
  (WAB) 214–16
WhatsApp 156
wheelchairs 64–5, 147, 157
Whitworth, A. 134
Wolfson Neurorehabilitation
  Centre 188, 213
word finding difficulties
  (WFD) 31–2, 161–2, 103,
  190–1
word lists 30
words for therapy 137
work: return to 33–6; talking
  about 194–5
working memory
  (WM) 88, 91, 105, 135;
  definition 243
World Health Organisation
  (WHO): COVID-19
  pandemic 93; International
  Classification of Functioning,
  Disability and Health (ICF)
  16, 20, 30, 72–4, 104, 128
writing 138–9, 157

yoga 179

For Product Safety Concerns and Information please contact our EU representative GPSR@taylorandfrancis.com
Taylor & Francis Verlag GmbH, Kaufingerstraße 24, 80331 München, Germany

www.ingramcontent.com/pod-product-compliance
Lightning Source LLC
Chambersburg PA
CBHW060558230426
4367OCB00011B/1873